INSTRUCTOR'S MANUAL AND GUIDELINES FOR

# Holistic Nursing

## *A Handbook for Practice*

FOURTH EDITION

**Barbara Montgomery Dossey, RN, PhD, HNC, FAAN**
Director
Holistic Nursing Consultants
Santa Fe, New Mexico

**Lynn Keegan, RN, PhD, HNC, FAAN**
Director
Holistic Nursing Consultants
Port Angeles, Washington

**Cathie E. Guzzetta, RN, PhD, HNC, FAAN**
Nursing Research Consultant
Children's Medical Center of Dallas
Director
Holistic Nursing Consultants
Dallas, Texas

Endorsed by the American Holistic Nurses' Association

JONES AND BARTLETT PUBLISHERS
*Sudbury, Massachusetts*
BOSTON TORONTO LONDON SINGAPORE

*World Headquarters*
Jones and Bartlett Publishers
40 Tall Pine Drive
Sudbury, MA 01776
978-443-5000
info@jbpub.com
www.jbpub.com

Jones and Bartlett Publishers
Canada
2406 Nikanna Road
Mississauga, ON L5C 2W6
CANADA

Jones and Bartlett Publishers
International
Barb House, Barb Mews
London W6 7PA
UK



The author has made every effort to ensure the accuracy of the information herein. However, appropriate information sources should be consulted, especially for new or unfamiliar procedures. It is the responsibility of every practitioner to evaluate the appropriateness of a particular opinion in the context of actual clinical situations and with due considerations to new developments. The authors, editors, and the publisher cannot be held responsible for any typographical or other errors found in this book.

Production Credits
Acquisitions Editor: Kevin Sullivan
Production Manager: Amy Rose
Editorial Assistant: Amy Sibley
Production Assistant: Tracey Chapman
Marketing Manager: Ed McKenna
Manufacturing Buyer: Amy Bacus
Composition: Northeast Compositors, Inc.
Cover Design: Anne Spencer
Printing and Binding: Malloy, Inc.
Cover Printing: Malloy, Inc.

*Printed in the United States of America*
08 07 06 05 04 10 9 8 7 6 5 4 3 2 1

# Table of Contents

# Introduction

A course in holistic nursing, integrating the art and science of caring and healing, is extraordinary, rewarding, and fulfilling. This is a process course and requires that process strategies be used to present the different topics and modalities. For students to learn the dynamics of health promotion and healing, theoretical content must be presented both in lecture format and in experiential sessions. The course is an opportunity to help students realize what it means to live healthy and inspired lives. It is a journey with students to investigate the unity and relatedness of all aspects of living and dying; to awaken the healing potentials within self and others; and to develop and explore different strategies to strengthen the whole person. We invite you and your students to undertake and explore the translation of healing by asking four significant questions:

1. What do you know about the meaning of healing?
2. What can you do each day to facilitate healing in yourself?
3. What is the essence of being a nurse healer?
4. What can you do to enhance your presence of being a nurse healer?

This Instructor's Manual has been developed to assist in the facilitation and integration of holistic principles. We have offered many strategies. Be creative and add your own personal style to these strategies, guidelines, and suggestions. This course exposes students to the experience of presence and healing. It teaches students different aspects of how to "walk the talk" of holism. The textbook content, chapter format, and teaching methods are designed to nurture the individual student's body, mind, and spirit. The various teaching methods enhance the student's creativity. This leads to sharing and healing of self and sharing of ways to integrate these dimensions into all aspects of one's being. This class experience builds trust in self as well as knowledge of how to create a healing community with colleagues.

## INTEGRATION OF HEALING RITUALS

We encourage the integration of rituals and the creative arts in each class as a way of connecting with the sacred life force. Rituals allow for a noninterfering attention to being present in the moment that allows natural healing to flow. They are essential strategies for professional and personal integration of holistic principles. When students are exposed to rituals and the creative arts that evoke presence and healing, this unique quality time, in class as well as outside of class requirements, will empower them to transfer this experience to clinical practice and other areas of their lives. It will also assist them in future work situations to care for self and to support colleagues in their healing.

The rituals may be a simple opening guided relaxation and imagery exercise (10–15 minutes) incorporating music or a longer experiential session incorporating clay modeling, mask making, or mandala drawing. An important aspect of inner work in our fast-paced lives is to create a time for rituals that have specific meaning. In creating a healing ritual, there are no absolute rules that should be followed. One guideline is that a ritual should have a structure—a beginning, a middle, and an end.

Any ritual has three phases. The first phase of a ritual, the *separation phase*, is a symbolic act of breaking away from life's busy activities. In the second phase of a ritual, the *transition phase*, we can more easily identify areas in our lives that need attention. Finally, in the last phase of a ritual, the *return phase*, we reenter real life.

## INSTRUCTOR'S ROLE

The instructor must be committed to health promotion and holistic principles, and must be experienced with and use complementary therapies in clinical practice and personal life.

Develop your role as facilitator and coach in integrating complementary healing modalities with traditional modalities in the classroom, clinical settings, and daily living. Encourage the students to focus on self-care as an important dimension of holistic nursing. Be creative in classroom presentations, discussion, and experiential activities.

**Style.** Use different teaching techniques and complementary modalities that allow your passion for caring and healing to emerge. Use your creative gifts. Which arts speak to you? How do you respond to music, art, paintings, weaving, sculpting, and so on?

**Coaching Students.** To assist students in understanding and integrating the content, coach students in how to teach the experiential sessions in a chosen class presentation. Students will present their ideas to the instructor. The instructor will coach students in how to guide classmates in different experiential exercises on a selected topic.

**Guest Speakers.** You are encouraged to invite different speakers from the community who can bring relevance to different topics as well as to the integration of different healing modalities. Ask these experts to incorporate the use of the healing arts in their presentations if appropriate. Provide the speaker with theoretical, clinical, and personal objectives from the specific textbook chapter if the topic is to be presented by a guest lecturer.

**Audiovisual Aids.** Incorporate PowerPoint, slides, overhead projections, videos, and music to enhance the material. Arrange for a screen, projector (for PowerPoint or slides), and pointer; audiocassette recorder or CD player for playing music, or a videocassette recorder; and television for showing videos. Even if you are in a small classroom, the use of a microphone is encouraged. This allows the person leading the guided relaxation and imagery exercises to speak in a relaxed manner and not to strain the voice to be heard over background music. It also helps students learn how to use their voices effectively as a therapeutic instrument of healing.

**Healing Environment.** Be creative with your classroom. Invite students to bring floor pillows for sitting for experiential exercises. Hang colorful posters, flowers, and plants and consider providing running water that flows into a small open reservoir or container (small, inexpensive pumps and containers can be found at garden nurseries). You can even hold some of your classes out in nature for sharing circles, walking meditation, etc. Encourage students to be tuned into the natural rhythms and cycles of nature. Use naturally occurring events in nature (the changing seasons, planting seeds, flowering, going into hibernation, etc.) as metaphors in teaching situations and in the sharing of personal stories in healing circles.

**Supplies for Healing Rituals.** Some elements and objects that can be used in rituals are imagination, candles, music, drums, altar or sacred space, circles, masks, songs, incense, healing symbols, totems, fetishes, poetry, chants, feathers, colored yarns, crayons, colored construction paper, pictures, stories, talking sticks, flowers, water, earth elements, clay, and other art supplies. Gather these art supplies and various healing objects as seen in Figures 1 and 2. Place supplies in baskets for easy transport to class as well as for storage between classes.

**Healing Tapestry.** Creation of a healing tapestry is a unique process experience and helps students to understand more quickly the qualities of recognizing and facilitating healing in self and others. You may wish to have students create a healing tapestry and add different qualities of healing in each class throughout the course. This tapestry can also be adapted for use with another topic discussed in the course. The steps for creating a healing tapestry are found in Appendix A and are seen in Figures 3 and 4. An adaptation to the healing tapestry exercise is shown in Figure 5. A guided imagery script that incorporates qualities of healing is given in Appendix B.

**Sharing Circles.** Have students read Chapter 10, "The Nurse As an Instrument of Healing," in preparation for the third class session. This chapter focuses on essential steps in healing, presence, and the art of guiding. It prepares students for introduction to sharing circles.

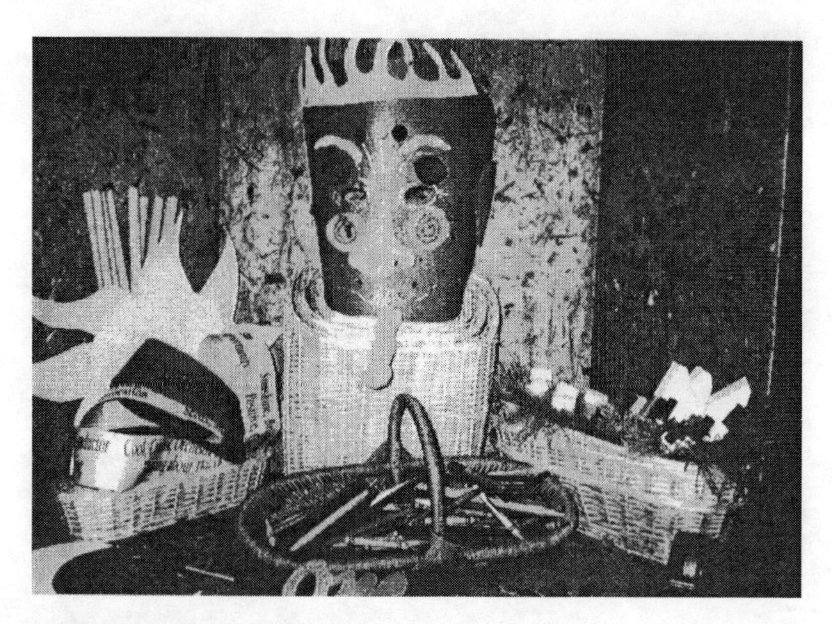

**Figure 1** Art Supplies for Healing Rituals

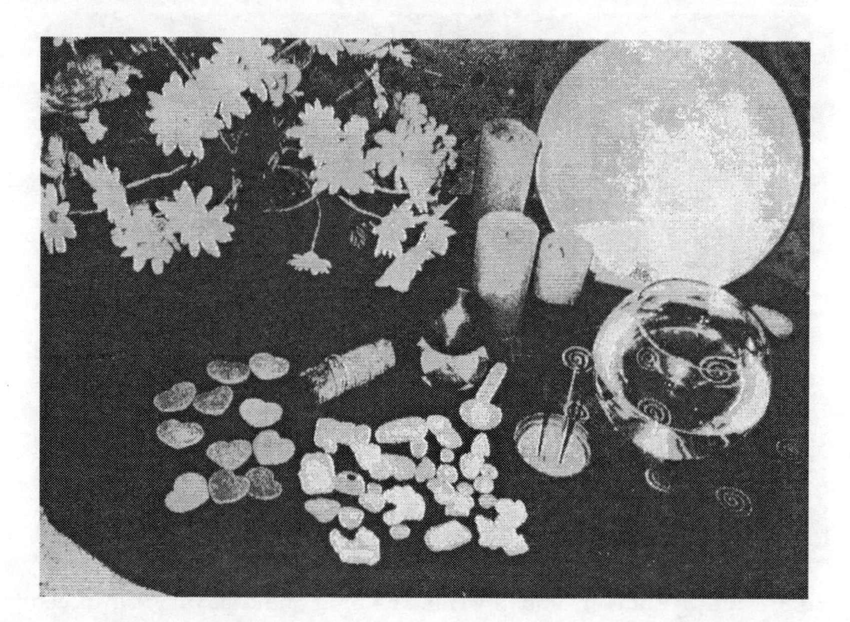

**Figure 2** Objects for Healing Rituals

Sharing circles last 15 to 20 minutes or longer and include groups of three to six students; they are held each class session. These sharing circles provide opportunities to recount healing moments and discuss any personal issues that are in need of healing. Sharing circles encourage the "listening council process."

Ask students to be mindful of the dialogue process and active listening. Encourage students to speak "from the heart." When the skills

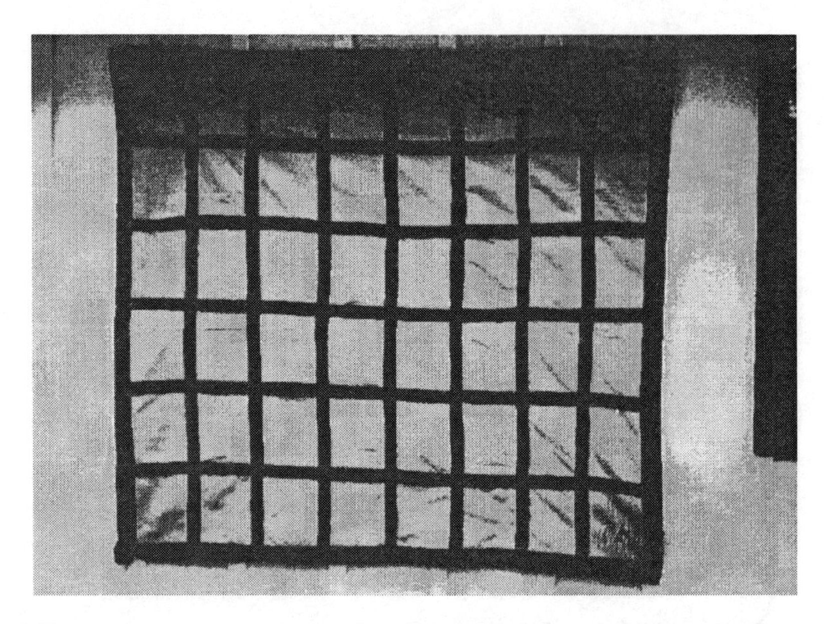

**Figure 3** Blank Tapestry

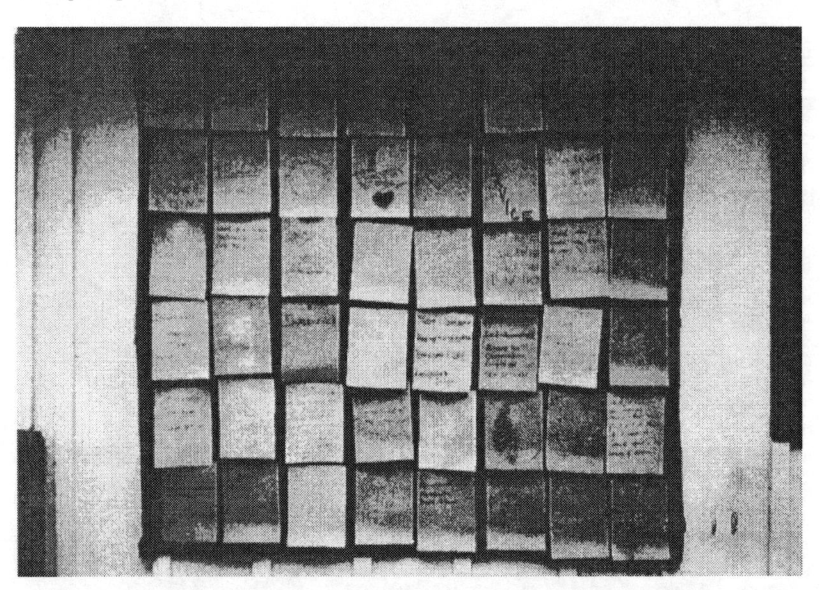

**Figure 4** Healing Tapestry. Students have written healing qualities and drawn healing images and symbols on different pieces of colored construction paper. These are attached to the blank felt tapestry by placing adhersive-backed male Velcro dots on the back of the paper; these dots easily adhere to an open square on the felt tapestry (see Appendix A for details).

---

of speaking with intention are developed, an individual is able to be present and avoid superficial comments. To encourage reflection, suggest that students have a moment of silence before sharing. This is not a time for "psychoanalyzing" each other, but a time to practice presence in the moment and speaking from a place of authentic sharing. This helps in keeping the dialogue open, because students learn to build trust and concern for self and others.

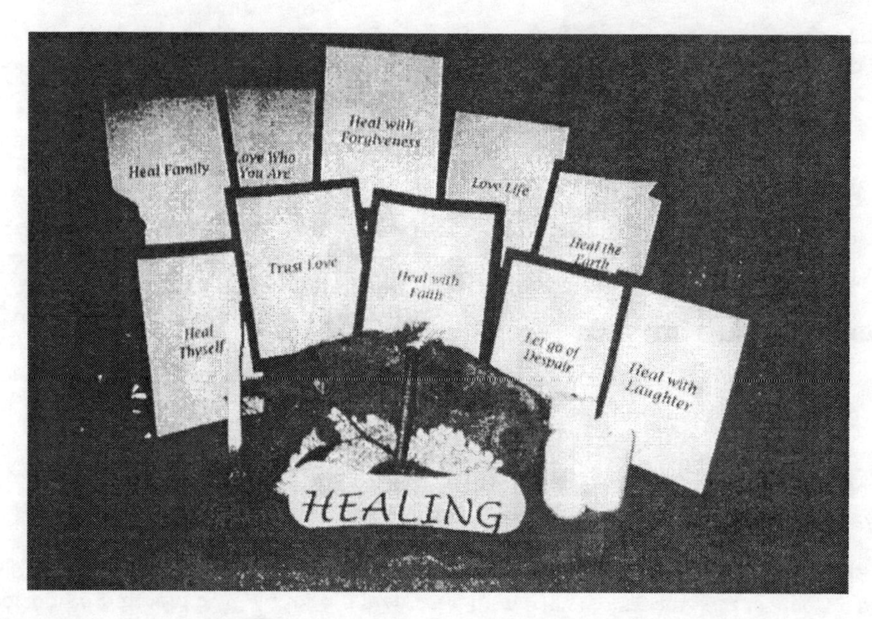


**Figure 5** Recognizing Healing Qualities. Students have combined art and healing objects as part of a class presentation

---

A talking stick or healing object may be used by a person before talking. Before speaking, a person picks up a talking stick or a healing object and then speaks with intention. Only the person with the talking stick or healing object in his or her hand speaks. As students learn to be present with self, to hear stories of healing, joy, or deep pain, and to share the struggles and triumphs of each individual's own journey, they learn to validate the importance of caring and healing moments.

## STUDENT'S ROLE

**Class Session Topic(s).** Read chapter(s) and complete homework assignment(s) before each class. Come to class with an openness to develop new skills, to actively participate, and to increase understanding of what is meant by "allowing healing presence into each moment."

**Class Presentation.** Active participation is essential. Students will choose a group and a topic, and each group will give a 2-hour class presentation. This group will develop, plan, and prepare a handout and case study along with an experiential session related to the topic. This session will also require a practice and rehearsal outside of class. If a guest speaker is to be part of this class presentation, the students will work with the instructor to invite the best-qualified person to present.

**Support Group Meetings.** Attend two different support group meetings. Write a short report on each meeting that reflects integration of health belief model, stages of change theory (Chapter 3), holistic theory and strategies, and personal experiences (in all chapters).

**Circle of Human Potential Self-Assessments.** Complete these self-assessments (Chapter 15) at the beginning and end of the course.

**Mindfulness Practice.** Begin a practice of mindfulness (10 minutes each day). This practice may include strategies such as relaxation, imagery, music, prayer, or meditation, or movement such as a walking meditation. Daily practice sessions may begin with "The part of me that is most in need of healing is . . ." or "The part of my life that I want to develop or to grow in is . . ." See Appendix C for student guidelines.

**Journaling.** Begin keeping a journal (5 minutes each day). Students are encouraged to use the "Nurse Healer Reflections" section at the end of the assigned chapter(s) as a guide for journal entries. Students may also incorporate any insights, emotions, changes in stress level, attitudes, healthier behaviors, difficulties in daily practice, and so on. See Appendix D for student guidelines.

## CHAPTER PREPARATION AND PRESENTATION

We recommend a four-stage process, as follows.

**Process Exercise/Vision of Healing.** Read the process exercise entitled "Vision of Healing" preceding each chapter for class discussion. What rings as truth when you read? Highlight these areas. Connect the process exercise with the "Vision of Healing" content. If two or more chapters are to be presented in the same class session, integrate the different process exercises throughout the class. Use the guidelines given or develop a new ritual. Begin each class with an experiential exercise or a ritual that sets the stage and tone to evoke healing and presence. It will also help students gain a deeper understanding of how to create sacred space within oneself and in the moment.

**Chapter Objectives.** Be creative about how chapter objectives are met. The theoretical objectives can be met by instructor presentation, guest lecturer, use of videos, experiential sessions, and other assigned activities. The clinical area objectives can be met in or out of the classroom in different community support group sessions, student group presentations, and experiential sessions. The personal objectives can be met by class participation, mindfulness practice, and journaling.

**Quick Chapter Read-Through.** Get an overall feel for chapter definitions and chapter content. Identify major themes you wish to present and highlight these areas.

**Class Session Preparation.** Allow 1 hour for structured presentation and 2 hours for experiential and sharing circles. Be flexible with these times depending on what the topic is and whether there will be guest speakers, videos, or a student group presentation. Student presentations begin with Session 6. Assist and coach students in developing their chosen topics and in the most effective way to present the subject and experiential session.

## CLOSING COURSE RITUAL

This process course will seem incomplete without a closing ritual. Invite a group of students to join you in creating a special closing healing celebration ritual. This may include the sharing of food and beverages. As the course evolves over the semester, you and the students will know exactly how to bring closure to the course.

## AFTERWORD

We hope that this Instructor's Manual will help you and your students derive a rewarding experience from the textbook. If you would like to share your suggestions and creative endeavors regarding course curriculum and healing rituals for future editions of this Instructor's Manual and textbook, we would enjoy hearing from you.* We support and applaud you for creating this learning opportunity for students. Best wishes in your healing journey, work, and life.

*Barbara Montgomery Dossey*
*Lynn Keegan*
*Cathie E. Guzzetta*

---

*Send suggestions, course descriptions, and healing rituals to: Jones and Bartlett Publishers, 40 Tall Pine Drive, Sudbury, Massachusetts 01776.

# Sample Course Description

## COURSE TITLE

FOUNDATIONS OF HOLISTIC NURSING

## COURSE CREDIT

3 Credits

## HOURS

45 theoretical and experiential hours

## CURRICULUM PLACEMENT

Undergraduate junior or senior course elective
Graduate course elective

## CATALOGUE DESCRIPTION

Seminar discussion of holistic practice and interventions, demonstration and/or experiential sessions to facilitate understanding of a holistic perspective in nursing practice and daily living. This course is specifically designed to help students comprehend the meaning of a holistic perspective for theoretical development, practice, and daily life.

## CONCEPTUAL FRAMEWORK

The course is built around the dimensions that comprise the practice of holistic nursing: bio-psycho-social-spiritual theory, interventions, and research; nurse-focused, client/patient-focused, and family/significant others-focused concepts of caring/healing and health promotion; experiential interventions and strategies to enhance effective communication with self and others.

## COURSE OBJECTIVES

At the completion of this course, the student will be able to

- discuss the holistic dimension as a world view from a processional and personal perspective
- examine the purpose of holistic principles from a bio-psycho-social-spiritual perspective
- analyze the congruence of the holistic perspective with nursing's humanistic base
- evaluate the application of holistic modalities in clinical practice and daily life
- discuss the implementation of holistically oriented research findings into clinical practice and daily life
- integrate nursing theory and experiences from a holistic perspective

## OUTLINE

Holistic Nursing Practice; Transpersonal Human Caring and Healing; Nursing Theory in Holistic Nursing Practice; The Art of Holistic Nursing and the Human Health Experience; The Psychophysiology of Bodymind Healing; Spirituality and Health; Energetic Healing; Holistic Ethics; Holistic Nursing Research; The Nurse As an Instrument of Healing; Therapeutic Communication: The Art of Helping; Environment; Cultural Diversity and Care; The Holistic Caring Process; Self-Assessments: Facilitating Healing in Self and Others; Cognitive Therapy; Self-Reflection: Consulting the Truth Within; Nutrition; Exercise and Movement; Humor, Laughter, and Play: Maintaining Balance in a Serious World; Relaxation: The First Step to Restore, Renew, and Self-Heal; Imagery: Awakening the Inner Healer; Music Therapy: Hearing the Melody of the Soul; Touch: Connecting with the Healing Power; Relationships; Dying in Peace; Weight Management Counseling; Smoking Cessation: Freedom from Risk; Addiction and Recovery Counseling; Incest and Child Sexual Abuse Counseling; Aromatherapy; Relationship-Centered Care and Healing Initiative in a Community Hospital; Exploring Integrative Medicine and the Healing Environment: The Story of a Large Urban Acute Care Hospital.

## TEACHING AND LEARNING STRATEGIES*

- Seminar (theory, experiential sessions, PowerPoint slides, overhead projections, videos, handouts)
- In class: group presentation and class participation
- Out of class: two support group meetings of choice (12-step programs, I Can Cope, HIV/AIDS, weight management, etc.); self-assessments; mindfulness practice (10 minutes a day); and journaling (5 minutes a day)
- Guest speakers (e.g., practitioners of Therapeutic Touch, biofeedback, art, music, movement, and/or healers from different cultures, etc.)

## EVALUATION METHODS†

50% Group presentation, which includes case study, handout, and experiential session that integrates one or more holistic interventions. Integration of four current journal articles related to class topic include at least one research article and at least one article on related area of interest.

20% Attendance at two different support group meetings. Short written report on each meeting that reflects integration of health belief model, stages of change theory, holistic theory and strategies, and personal experiences.

10% Complete Circle of Human Potential self-assessments at beginning and end of course.

20% Mindfulness practice (10 minutes a day); journaling (5 minutes a day).

## REQUIRED TEXT

B. M. Dossey, L. Keegan, and C. E. Guzzetta. *Holistic Nursing: A Handbook for Practice*, 4th ed. (Sudbury, MA: Jones and Bartlett, 2004).

## INSTRUCTOR'S MANUAL

B. Dossey, L. Keegan, and C. Guzzetta. *Instructor's Manual and Guidelines for Holistic Nursing: A Handbook for Practice*, 4th ed. (Sudbury, MA: Jones and Bartlett, 2004).

*The following teaching and learning strategies apply if this course and textbook are used in a university setting as part of an undergraduate or graduate elective. If this course is taught outside of a university setting or is used as a home study course, these teaching and learning strategies can be supportive learning experiences and are suggested for the student to consider in home study.

†Suggested evaluation method if this course and textbook are used in a university setting as part of an undergraduate or graduate elective. If this course is to be taught outside of a university setting, see instructions for home study course in "Information for Continuing Education and Home Study."

# Sample Course Outline

**SESSION 1**

Course introduction and course overview (1 hour).

Discuss that this is a process course and thus requires active participation. Stress importance of reading class assignment before coming to class. Give course requirements and guidelines for mindfulness practice and for journaling. Student presentations begin with Session 6. Session 6–13 topics will be student presentations. Introduce students to the five core values of the textbook.

*Core Value 1:* Holistic Philosophy, Theories, and Ethics
*Core Value 2:* Holistic Education and Research
*Core Value 3:* Holistic Nurse Self-Care
*Core Value 4:* Holistic Communication, Therapeutic Environment, and Cultural Diversity
*Core Value 5:* Holistic Caring Process

*Process Exercise No. 15*

Chapter 15. Self-Assessments: Facilitating Healing in Self and Others
Complete Self-Assessments (Chapter 15)
Review AHNA Standards of Holistic Nursing (Chapter 1, Appendix 1–A)

**SESSION 2**

*Process Exercises Nos. 1, 2, and 6*

Chapter 1. Holistic Nursing Practice
Chapter 2. Transpersonal Human Caring and Healing
Chapter 6. The Psychophysiology of Bodymind Healing

**SESSION 3**

*Process Exercises Nos. 7, 10, and 17*

Chapter 7. Spirituality and Health
Chapter 10. The Nurse As an Instrument of Healing
Chapter 17. Self-Reflection: Consulting the Truth Within
Appendix A (Instructor's Manual): Guidelines for Creating a Healing Tapestry
Appendix B (Instructor's Manual): Script: Creating a Healing Tapestry

**SESSION 4**

*Process Exercises Nos. 4, 5, and 9*

Chapter 4. Nursing Theory in Holistic Nursing Practice
Chapter 5. Holistic Ethics
Chapter 9. Holistic Nursing Research

**SESSION 5**

*Process Exercises Nos. 8 and 24*

Chapter 8. Energetic Healing
Chapter 24. Touch: Connecting with the Healing Power

**STUDENT PRESENTATIONS BEGIN WITH SESSION 6**

**SESSION 6**

*Process Exercises Nos. 11, 13, and 14*

Chapter 11. Therapeutic Communication: The Art of Helping
Chapter 13. Cultural Diversity and Care
Chapter 14. The Holistic Caring Process

**SESSION 7**

*Process Exercises Nos. 16 and 20*

Chapter 16. Cognitive Therapy
Chapter 20. Humor, Laughter, and Play: Maintaining Balance in a Serious World

**SESSION 8**

*Process Exercises Nos. 21 and 23*

Chapter 21. Relaxation: The First Step to Restore, Renew, and Self-Heal
Chapter 23. Music Therapy: Hearing the Melody of the Soul

**SESSION 9**

***Process Exercises Nos. 22 and 31***

Chapter 22. Imagery: Awakening the Inner Healer
Chapter 31. Aromatherapy

**SESSION 10**

***Process Exercises Nos. 12***

Chapter 12. Environment

**SESSION 11**

***Process Exercise No. 26***

Chapter 26. Dying in Peace

**SESSION 12**

***Process Exercises Nos. 3, 28, and 29***

Chapter 3. The Art of Holistic Nursing and the Human Health Experience
Chapter 28. Smoking Cessation: Freedom from Risk
Chapter 29. Addiciton and Recovery Counseling

**SESSION 13**

***Process Exercises Nos. 18, 19, and 27***

Chapter 18. Nutrition
Chapter 19. Exercise and Movement
Chapter 27. Weight Management Counseling

**SESSION 14**

***Process Exercises Nos. 25 and 30***

Chapter 25. Relationships
Chapter 30. Incest and Child Sexual Abuse Counseling

**SESSION 15**

***Process Exercises Nos. 32 and 33***

Chapter 32. Relationships-Centered Care and Healing Initiative in a Community Hospital
Chapter 33. Exploring Integrative Medicine and the Healing Environment: The Story of a Large Urban Acute Care Hospital

**CLOSING RITUAL AND CELEBRATION**

# Information for Continuing Education and Home Study

The American Holistic Nurses' Association (AHNA) provides continuing education (CE) credit when this textbook is used as a course or course segment(s) outside of a university setting (see Options 1, 2, 3, and 4), and when it is used in home study.

The AHNA is accredited as a provider of continuing education in nursing by the Commission of Accreditation of the American Nurses Credentialing Center.

To obtain information on holistic nursing course or course segments CE, CE fee, and CE certificates, contact:

Education Administrator
American Holistic Nurses' Association
P.O. Box 2130
Flagstaff, AZ 86003-2130
Attn: Home Study Materials
Phone: (800) 278-AHNA or (520) 526-2196
Fax: (520) 526-2752
E-Mail: education@AHNA.org

The course Foundations of Holistic Nursing can be taught as a course or course segment(s) outside a university setting. The course or course segment(s) (see Options 1, 2, 3, and 4) must be taught and developed by a holistic nurse with a minimum of a baccalaureate degree who has applied and been accepted by AHNA as a "Lead Instructor." An AHNA Lead Instructor may sponsor the following:

- a course or course segment(s) on holistic nursing practice as part of an independent practice
- a course or course segment(s) on holistic nursing practice for a hospital/medical center nursing education development and research department
- a course or course segment(s) on holistic nursing practice for a community continuing education program such as a winter, spring, summer, or fall series.

## AHNA HOME STUDY COURSE: HOLISTIC NURSING

*AHNA Holistic Nursing: A Handbook for Practice*, 4th Edition. By B. M. Dossey, L. Keegan, and C. E. Guzzetta (Sudbury, MA: Jones and Bartlett, 2004). ISBN: 0-7637-3183-8. Phone: 1-800-638-8437.

The textbook *Holistic Nursing: A Handbook for Practice* can be used as an AHNA home study course. You can either take one or more segments or the whole package. See the instructions below on Options 1, 2, 3, and 4. A total of 54 contact hours (CE) for home study can be obtained by completing a home study log and taking the final examination of 100 questions. A score of 70 percent or higher is required to receive the AHNA CE credit. The workbook study log and final examination for this AHNA home study course can be obtained from the AHNA. Contact the AHNA for information regarding the AHNA home study course fee. This AHNA home study course can be used to meet the CE requirement toward holistic nursing certification or recertification as evidence of continuing education in holistic nursing.

To receive AHNA home study course CE credit (up to 54 contact hours) for the course based on *Holistic Nursing: A Handbook for Practice*, complete the following steps:

1. Purchase a copy of *Holistic Nursing: A Handbook for Practice, 4th Edition* from Jones and Bartlett Publishers or from a local bookstore.
2. Contact the AHNA for information on the course fee. Write the AHNA to receive the workbook log, final examination, and final examination answer sheet.
   - Complete the AHNA home study course participant form for *Holistic Nursing: A Handbook for Practice*.

## HOLISTIC NURSING COURSE OR HOME STUDY SEGMENT(S) DESCRIPTIONS

**Lead Teacher Course/ Course Segment(s):** **Foundations of Holistic Nursing.** Course/course segment(s) based on the textbook *Holistic Nursing: A Handbook for Practice*, 4th ed. B. M. Dossey, L. Keegan, and C. E. Guzzetta (Sudbury, MA: Jones and Bartlett, 2004) and the accompanying Instructor's Manual.

**OPTION 1:** **Foundations of Holistic Nursing.** (See Instructor's Manual.) All 15 sessions (3 hours each)

**Contact Hours Awarded:** 54.0 contact hours

**OPTION 2:** **Foundations of Holistic Nursing.** (See Instructor's Manual.) Any 6-topic combination of 3-hour course segment(s) (Example: Holistic Nursing, Nurse as an Instrument of Healing, Relaxation, Imagery, Music Therapy, and Touch)

**Contact Hours Awarded:** 21.6 contact hours

**OPTION 3:** **Foundations of Holistic Nursing.** (See Instructor's Manual.) Any 2-topic combination of 3-hour course segment(s) (Example: Relaxation and Imagery)

**Contact Hours Awarded:** 7.2 Contact Hours

**OPTION 4:** **Foundations of Holistic Nursing.** (See Instructor's Manual.) Any 3-hour course segment (Example: Imagery)

**Contact Hours Awarded:** 3.6 contact hours

- Send the home study course fee (to be paid by money order or credit card; fee is nonrefundable) to the AHNA.

3. After you receive the AHNA home study course workbook log, final examination, and final examination answer sheet for *Holistic Nursing: A Handbook for Practice*, do the following:
   - Complete the workbook log.
   - Take the final examination and enter your correct answers on the final examination answer sheet using a no. 2 lead pencil as instructed. *This is the only answer sheet that will be used for scoring your exam.*
   - Send the AHNA your worksheet log and final examination answer sheet.

If you successfully pass the final examination with a score of 70 percent or higher, you will receive your AHNA home study course certificate (up to 54 contact hours) within 6 weeks.

Keep a copy of all AHNA home study course records. Mail the above items to

AHNA Continuing Education
Ameican Holistic Nurses' Association
P.O. Box 2130
Flagstaff, AZ 86003-2130
Attn: Home Study Materials

If you have questions, call, fax, or e-mail the AHNA at

Phone: (800) 278-AHNA
Fax: (520) 528-2752
E-mail: education@AHNA.org

## HOLISTIC NURSING CERTIFICATION

*Holistic Nursing: A Handbook for Practice* can be used along with the AHNA *Core Curriculum for Holistic Nursing* to prepare for the American Holistic Nurses' Certification Corporation (AHNCC) certification examination. For AHNCC information on both basic and advanced certification, contact

American Holistic Nurses' Certification Corporation
5102 Ganymede Drive
Austin, TX 78727
E-mail: ahncc@HASH.net

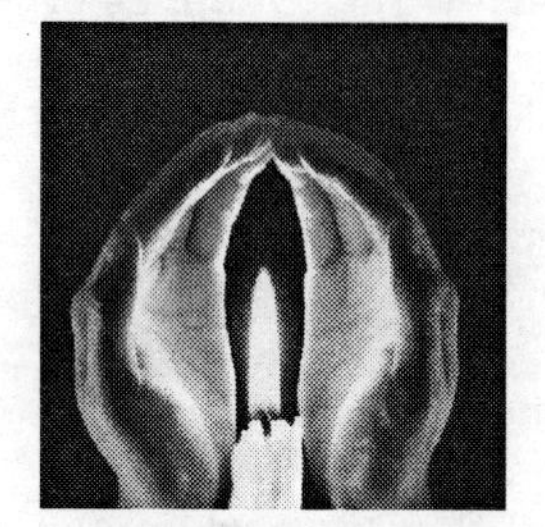

# CORE VALUE 1

# Holistic Philosophy, Theories, and Ethics

## Chapter 1

## Holistic Nursing Practice

### CHAPTER OBJECTIVES

Refer to chapter for specific theoretical, clinical, and personal objectives. These will provide guidelines for the integration of objectives in class presentation, experiential sessions, and student homework assignments.

### CHAPTER OVERVIEW

Two major challenges have emerged in nursing. The first challenge is to integrate the concepts of technology, mind, and spirit into nursing practice. The second challenge is to create models for health care that guide the healing of self and others. Holistic nursing is the most complete way to conceptualize and practice professional nursing.

### PROCESS EXERCISE NO. 1

(15-minute opening experiential session using music and healing objects if desired.)

#### Vision of Healing: Exploring Life's Meaning

As we explore meaning and purpose, we are able to access those events that are most important as well as more easily identify passions in life. Meanings are individual and personal. As we explore our personal experience with daily events, we move closer to a deeper understanding of holism.

Begin with a guided relaxation exercise (5 minutes) and gradually fade in music of choice. Suggest to students that they can close their eyes or leave their eyes open. Ask students who leave their eyes open to focus on a spot several feet in front of them. This allows for a greater ease in following the relaxation and imagery suggestions and reflective experience.

Using techniques for empowering relaxation and imagery scripts (see Chapters 21 and 22), gently weave into a guided imagery exercise reflective questions from the Spiritual Assessment Tool (Exhibit 7-3) such as: What gives your life meaning and purpose? What are your personal strengths? Do you ever feel at some level a connection with the world or universe? Add three to five more reflective questions under each of the categories (in boldface in the exhibit). Bring closure to the imagery process.

With soft music still playing, invite students to record in a personal journal (3 to 5 minutes) any images, process questions and answers, or insight gained. Ask students to bring personal closure to this process. Gradually fade music out. Engage students in a gentle stretching exercise before the theory session begins.

## KEY CONCEPTS: THEORY AND RESEARCH

(1-hour presentation)
**OPTIONAL: GUEST SPEAKER(S) AND VIDEO(S)**

**Guest Speaker(s):** Invite a nurse who integrates holistic modalities in clinical practice or a panel of nurses in different practice settings that are guided in practice by a bio-psycho-social-spiritual model. Provide guest speaker(s) with the Instructor's Manual suggestions so the speaker(s) can become familiar with the students' assignment before class.

**Video(s):** Show a video of a practitioner describing and demonstrating one or more holistic modalities (rent from media catalogue or purchase for school video library). Following the video presentation, ask students for their reactions and comments. Discuss the video and answer questions.

**Definitions:** Review definitions and incorporate into presentation.

## HOLISM

**Natural Systems Theory:** Review holism and natural systems theory (Figure 1–1). Explain the Western, allopathic medical model (Table 1–1) that has been used for the last 150 years in diagnosis and treatment of disease. Discuss how this model is incomplete as the remaining topics in this section are integrated. Contrast the allopathic and holistic models of care.

**Bio-Psycho-Social-Spiritual Model:** Explore the components of a bio-psycho-social-spiritual model (Figure 1–2) and its implications for holistic nursing and healing. Discuss the interdependence and the interrelatedness of all parts.

## HOLISTIC NURSING

**Description of Holistic Nursing:** Review the definition of holistic nursing.

**Standards of Holistic Nursing Practice:** Review the interrelationship of the five core values (Figure 1–3) contained in the American Holistic Nurses' Association Standards of Holistic Nursing Practice. Explore the definitions and action statements in each core value (Appendix 1–A).

**Eras of Medicine:** Review the dynamics of the eras of medicine (Figure 1–4 and Table 1–2). Focus on states of consciousness and therapies in each—local states of consciousness in eras I and II, and nonlocal states of consciousness in era III. Discuss the "doing" and "not doing" approaches to healing (Figure 1–5). Discuss the NCCAM mission statement and research. Explore complementary therapies and their integration with traditional therapies. Contrast concepts and therapies of rational and paradoxical healing (Figure 1–6).

**Complementary and Alternative Therapies:** Discuss the role of the NCCAM research centers (Table 1–3) and how complementary and alternative therapies expand the strategies that nurses can employ independently to provide holistic, body-mind-spirit care (Exhibit 1–1).

**Relationship-Centered Care:** Review the philosophy of relationship-centered care and its three components: patient-practitioner relationship, community-practitioner relationship, and practitioner-practitioner relationship (Tables 1–4, 1–5, and 1–6).

## EXPERIENTIAL EXERCISES

(2 hours. Incorporation of sharing circles and experiential exercises is encouraged for class presentation.)

**Description of Holistic Nursing and the Standards for Holistic Nursing Practice:** Provide an overview of the AHNA Working Description of Holistic Nursing and the AHNA Standards of Holistic Nursing Practice (Appendix 1–A).

Have students work in five small groups. Each group will explore one core value of the AHNA Standards in depth. Allow time for each group to present comments and ideas from their assigned part of the AHNA Standards of Practice.

Ask students to share insights gained since Session 1 regarding increased awareness or importance of recognizing self-care concepts and the Circle of Human Potential (Chapter 15) each day.

**"Doing" and "Being" Therapies:** Present a case study that incorporates doing and being therapies. Have students share any personal stories or situations in which holistic modalities have been integrated, use of such modalities has been declined by client/patient or family, or allopathic physicians or nurses have blocked the use of holistic modalities in the clinical setting.

**Relationship-Centered Care:** Have students work in three groups. Each group will focus on one of the three components in relationship-centered care: patient-practitioner relationship, community-practitioner relationship, and practitioner-practitioner relationship. Have each group discuss and give examples of the areas of knowledge, skills, and values found in Tables 1–4, 1–5, and 1–6.

## DIRECTIONS FOR FUTURE RESEARCH

Have students choose one or more research questions as an area to explore; students should review the literature, identify research findings that could be utilized in practice, and/or postulate additional research questions or hypotheses. Consult with a nurse researcher to help develop a research study. Encourage students to begin collecting articles that can support further investigation.

## NURSE HEALER REFLECTIONS

Encourage students to use the chapter reflective questions as a guide to journal entries for exploring, understanding, and validating presence and healing.

# Chapter 2

# Transpersonal Human Caring and Healing

## CHAPTER OBJECTIVES

Refer to chapter for specific theoretical, clinical, and personal objectives. These will provide guidelines for the integration of objectives in class presentation, experiential sessions, and student homework assignments.

## CHAPTER OVERVIEW

Over the last 25 years, health care has been based on the allopathic, masculine model that has focused on the curing of symptoms. Individuals now recognize that both the allopathic approaches and complementary healing modalities are needed to stabilize or reverse disease and to improve quality of life.

## PROCESS EXERCISE NO. 2

(15-minute opening experiential session using music and healing objects if desired.)

### Vision of Healing: The Transpersonal Self

An important part of holistic nursing is connecting with inner healing resources. When nurses strive to explore their healing resources as a first step on the journey toward wholeness, they acknowledge inner wisdom essential to the healing process.

Begin with a guided relaxation exercise (5 minutes) and gradually fade in music of choice. Suggest to students that they can close their eyes or leave their eyes open. Ask students who leave their eyes open to focus on a spot several feet in front of them. This allows for a greater ease in following the relaxation and imagery suggestions and reflective experience.

Using techniques for empowering relaxation and imagery scripts (see Chapter 21 and 22), gently weave into a guided imagery exercise reflective questions of opening and being in the moment. Incorporate suggestions about being in right relationship and working in a healing system, and weave in concepts of "holding sacred space" as listed in Table 2–1.

With soft music still playing, invite your students to record in a personal journal (3 to 5 minutes) any images, process questions and answers, or insight gained. Ask students to bring personal closure to this process. Gradually fade music out. Engage students in a gentle stretching exercise before the theory session begins.

## KEY CONCEPTS: THEORY AND RESEARCH

(1-hour presentation)
**OPTIONAL: GUEST SPEAKER(S) AND VIDEO(S)**

**Guest Speaker(s):** Invite one or more nurses who have envisioned partnerships in clinical practice and have transformed parts of an established hospital system. Provide guest speaker(s) with the Instructor's Manual suggestions so the speaker(s) can become familiar with the students' assignment before class.

**Video(s):** Show a video of a nurse or a group of nurses describing and demonstrating the integration of holistic modalities and change in a traditional health care setting (rent from media catalogue or purchase for school video library). Following the video presentation, ask students for their reactions and comments. Discuss the video and answer questions.

**Definitions:** Review definitions and incorporate into presentation.

**Transpersonal Human Caring:** Develop the major themes identified in caring/healing research; review authenticity and healing awareness. Discuss the concepts of Watson's model of human caring.

**Healing: The Goal of Holistic Nursing:** Discuss the origin of the word *healing* and what it means.

**Healing as the Emergence of the Right Relationship:** Explore the concepts of wholeness and harmony, and the key principles in the right relationship and how this influences the nurse's and client's/patient's world view.

**Healing versus Curing:** Discuss the processes in healing and curing.

**Healing as an Outcome:** Explore "patterns of knowing" and how they can assist in the process of emergence in healing.

**Who or What the Healer Is:** Discuss the assumptions in healing and the way all healing emerges from within the totality of the unique body-mind-spirit of the patient.

**A True Healing Health Care System:** Identify the philosophy and interventions in a true healing health care system.

**Integration of the Masculine and the Feminine:** Review masculine and feminine qualities as they relate to a healing health care system and a sick care system.

**The Nurse as Healing Environment:** Explore the qualities that the nurse can use to enhance healing.

**The Wounded Healer:** Examine the components of a wounded healer and discuss recognition of one's woundedness as part of the journey of wholeness.

## EXPERIENTIAL EXERCISES

(2 hours. Incorporation of sharing circles and experiential exercises is encouraged for class presentation.)

**Transpersonal Human Caring:** Encourage students to identify areas of Watson's model of human caring and authenticity as well as healing awareness in their clinical practice and daily life.

**Healing as the Emergence of the Right Relationship:** Have students share clinical and personal experiences in which the process of harmony and a sense of authentic presence allowed the nurse to enter into a patient's personal story or experience.

**Healing versus Curing:** Have students give examples of case in which either healing or curing took place as well as cases in which they took place simultaneously.

**Healing as an Outcome:** Have students explore the use of the five senses to assist the nurse in the process of emergence in healing.

**A True Healing Health Care System:** Encourage students to determine whether a true healing health care system exists in their clinical setting and to identify some possible steps to enhance healing.

**Integration of the Masculine and the Feminine:** Have students discuss the differences between "getting the job done" and "holding sacred space" as listed in Table 2–1.

**The Nurse as Healing Environment:** Have students share examples of the strategies and awareness used to recognize aspects of being an instrument of healing.

**The Wounded Healer:** Encourage students to recognize the ongoing process of honoring one's woundedness as a necessary part of the journey toward wholeness.

## DIRECTIONS FOR FUTURE RESEARCH

Have students choose one or more research questions as an area to explore; students should review the literature, identify research findings that could be utilized in practice, and/or postulate additional research questions or hypotheses. Consult with a nurse researcher to help develop a research study. Encourage students to begin collecting articles that can support further investigation.

## NURSE HEALER REFLECTIONS

Encourage students to use the chapter reflective questions as a guide to journal entries for exploring, understanding, and validating presence and healing.

Chapter 3

# The Art of Holistic Nursing and the Human Health Experience

## CHAPTER OBJECTIVES

Refer to chapter for specific theoretical, clinical, and personal objectives. These will provide guidelines for the integration of objectives in class presentation, experiential sessions, and student homework assignments.

## CHAPTER OVERVIEW

As nurses explore the art of nursing and become more aware of the health-wellness-disease-illness that comprises the human health experience, they can more easily assist individuals in investigating the meaning of an acute crisis or illness. Values clarification, the health belief model, and the concept of stages of change are tools for understanding what complexities people confront and why certain behaviors exist. Knowledge of these concepts and theories can increase the nurse's awareness of the way in which values and beliefs affect each element of the motivational process and the stages of change. People must be motivated and engaged in the change process before they can begin to change behavior and to sustain maintenance behaviors that move them toward well-being.

## PROCESS EXERCISE NO. 3

(15-minute opening experiential session using music and other healing objects if desired.)

### Vision of Healing: Reawakening Spirit in Daily Life

When we exhibit hardiness characteristics, we can maximize our human potential. The three hardiness characteristics, referred to as the three Cs, are change, commitment, and control.

Begin with a guided relaxation exercise (5 minutes) and gradually fade in music of choice. Suggest to students that they can close their eyes or leave their eyes open. Ask students who leave their eyes open to focus on a spot several feet in front of them. This allows for a greater ease in following the relaxation and imagery suggestions and reflective experience.

Using techniques for empowering relaxation and imagery scripts (see Chapters 21 and 22), gently weave into a guided imagery exercise reflective questions about the hardiness characteristics known as the three Cs: change, commitment, control. Next weave into the imagery process reflective questions about how to increase levels of work spirit. Bring closure to the imagery process.

With soft music still playing, invite students to record in a personal journal (3 to 5 minutes) any images, process questions and answers, or insight gained. Ask students to bring personal closure to this process. Gradually fade music out. Engage students in a gentle stretching exercise before the theory session begins.

## KEY CONCEPTS: THEORY AND RESEARCH

(1-hour presentation)

**OPTIONAL: GUEST SPEAKER(S) AND VIDEO(S)**

**Guest Speaker(s):** Invite a nurse or nurses who direct a corporate wellness center. Provide guest speaker(s) with the Instructor's Manual suggestion so the speaker(s) can become familiar with the students' assignment before class.

**Video(s):** Show a video of a practitioner describing and demonstrating one or more folk medicine healing rituals (rent from media catalogue or purchase for school video library). Following video presentation, ask students for their reactions and comments. Discuss the video and answer questions.

**Definitions:** Review definitions and incorporate into presentation.

**The Art of Holistic Nursing:** Explore definitions and components of art and discuss how nurses are artists in their work. Examine how art arises out of the imagination and the six aspects of intuitive judgment.

**Aspects of the Human Health Experience:** Explore the relationship between health, wellness, disease, and illness by reviewing the definition of each. Discuss the importance of exploring the dynamics of each concept such as the actual or perceived function/dysfunction through the interactions of cognitive-affective dimensions that are developed in the text.

**Values Clarification and the Human Health Experience:** Review integrity as the first step in the art of nursing. Discuss the three steps in values clarification: choosing, prizing, and acting.

**Health Behaviors and the Human Health Experience:** Explore the use of *engagement* and *lack of engagement* as more appropriate terms than *compliance* and *noncompliance* for describing how people change or do not change health behaviors.

**Health Belief Model:** Discuss the major factors in determining a person's engagement in choosing new health behaviors. Examine the ways in which health beliefs, attitudes, and social support facilitate engagement. Review the four categories of the health belief model.

**Engagement:** Discuss use of the health belief model as a starting place for understanding the person's world view and assisting with the process of healing.

**Stages of Change in Addictive Behavior Patterns:** Discuss the five stages of change and the characteristics of each stage (Figure 3–1). Explore the dynamics of the change process and the most appropriate interventions at each stage (Exhibits 3–1 and 3–2).

**The Work Site and the Human Health Experience:** Explore the steps to take in developing a wellness program. Review circumstances that are known to block a person's motivated behavior.

## EXPERIENTIAL EXERCISES

(2 hours. Incorporation of sharing circles and experiential exercises is encouraged for class presentation.)

**The Art of Holistic Nursing:** Have students explore ways that they integrate art and are artists in their work. Ask them to give examples using the six aspects of intuitive judgment as a guideline.

**Aspects of the Human Health Experience:** Have students give clinical examples of health, wellness, disease, and illness and discuss the patient/family dynamics of the actual or perceived function/dysfunction through the interactions of cognitive-affective dimensions.

**Values Clarification:** Encourage students to become aware of their own differences in attitudes, beliefs, and values. Ask students to identify a goal or goals and to use the values clarification process—choosing, prizing, and acting—to change toward new ways of being.

Have students assess whether they have more attitudes and beliefs than values with regard to exercise, relaxation, and play. For example, a certain student believes that exercise is important for health and that it also serves to help manage stress and assists in achieving a sense of inner peace and harmony. However, this student has no exercise routine. Thus, this student has attitudes and beliefs about exercise rather than a value.

Have students use the above example to create a set of values for exercise (or another behavior that is desired) by using the three steps in the values clarification process.

## DIRECTIONS FOR FUTURE RESEARCH

Have students choose one or more research questions as an area to explore; students should review the literature, identify research findings that could be utilized in practice, and/or postulate additional research questions or hypotheses. Consult with a nurse researcher to help develop a research study. Encourage students to begin collecting articles that can support further investigation.

## NURSE HEALER REFLECTIONS

Encourage students to use the chapter reflective questions as a guide to journal entries for exploring, understanding, and validating presence and healing.

Chapter 4

# Nursing Theory in Holistic Nursing Practice

## CHAPTER OBJECTIVES

Refer to chapter for specific theoretical, clinical, and personal objectives. These will provide guidelines for the integration of objectives in class presentation, experiential sessions, and student homework assignments.

## CHAPTER OVERVIEW

This chapter explores the common ideas or concepts within all nursing theories—nursing, person, health, and environment. It addresses the need for theory and discusses how theory demands that the nurse reflect on this philosophy and on the way in which practice is working to achieve holistic ideas.

## PROCESS EXERCISE NO. 4

(15-minute opening experiential session using music and healing objects if desired.)

### Vision of Healing: Active Listening

Good listening is achieved by quieting the inner dialogue. Good listening has an enormous quality of nowness. Nowness is the ability to discard intellectualizations when the client heads in an unexpected direction. How often, when counseling a client who is intent on telling a part of his or her story, the nurse stops the flow of the study and brings the client back to a certain point; as a result, the client's insight may be blocked. Often we become too intent on a personal view of what we think should be happening, because we begin our own inner dialogue of analysis and intellectualization. As we increase this level of nowness, the client can also move to a state of nowness that allows an inner wisdom to merge. Questioning and listening that does not structure the answers, except minimally, is a great art.

Begin with a guided relaxation exercise (5 minutes) and gradually fade in music of choice. Suggest to students that they can close their eyes or leave their eyes open. Ask students who leave their eyes open to focus on a spot several feet in front of them. This allows for a greater ease in following the relaxation and imagery suggestions and reflective experience.

Using techniques for empowering relaxation and imagery scripts (see Chapters 21 and 22), gently weave reflective questions into a guided imagery exercise. Next, ask the students to remember a time recently when they were listening to another person's story. Can they recall really listening actively with intention? How did they feel when they knew that they were aware of being present with intention? Can they recall actively listening and really understanding someone, enjoying someone, learning something, or wanting to give help to someone?

Next, see if students can recall a time when they lapsed into pseudolistening as they were trying to meet the needs of others. Can they recall moments of pseudolistening which indicate that they were meeting personal needs and were not listening actively? Such instances might include

- keeping silent as you buy time to prepare your next remark
- listening to others so that they will listen to you
- listening only to specific information while ignoring the rest
- acting interested when you are not
- listening partially because you do not want to disappoint the other person
- listening in order not to be rejected
- searching for a person's weaknesses in order to take advantage of them
- identifying weak points in dialogue so that you can be stronger in your response

Next, have the students imagine that a very special person is listening actively to a story that they want to tell to facilitate their own healing. Guide students in the reflection as follows. Imagine that you are telling a story about a part of yourself that needs healing. If possible, can you be with your story and really live in what is happening right now, not avoiding it but letting it be? What is your body language as you experience yourself telling this story? How does it feel? What is conveyed? In telling this story, can you feel a greater acceptance of your own thoughts and emotions? Can you choose the most effective behaviors that may lead you toward greater inner peace and balance about the parts of yourself that can be healed in this moment?

With soft music still playing, invite students to record in a personal journal (3 to 5 minutes) any images, process questions and answers, or insight gained. Ask students to bring personal closure to this process. Gradually fade music out. Engage students in a gentle stretching exercise before the theory session begins.

## KEY CONCEPTS: THEORY AND RESEARCH

(1-hour presentation)

**OPTIONAL: GUEST SPEAKER(S) AND VIDEO(S)**

**Guest Speaker(s):** Invite a nurse who integrates holistic modalities in clinical practice or a panel of nurses in different practice settings that are guided in practice by a bio-psycho-social-spiritual model. Provide guest speaker(s) with the Instructor's Manual suggestions so the speaker(s) can become familiar with the students' reading assignment before class.

**Video(s):** Show a video of a practitioner describing and demonstrating one or more holistic modalities (rent from media catalogue or purchase for school video library). Following the video presentation, ask students for their reactions and comments. Discuss the video and answer questions.

**Definitions:** Review definitions and incorporate into presentation.

**Nursing Theory Defined:** Define nursing theory and the ideas and concepts common to all nursing theories.

**The Need for Theory:** Explore how nursing theory can guide nurses in the art and science of nursing. Discuss the five elements contained in the American Holistic Nurses' Association Description of Holistic Nursing: nursing knowledge, theories, expertise, intuition, and creativity; discuss how all these parts are essential for nurses to function in an ideal way.

**Theory Development:** Analyze the steps in theory development: description, explanation, prediction, and prescription. Discuss the specific nursing theories covered in the chapter that are most frequently used by holistic nurses: Florence Nightingale's theory, the theory of environmental adaptation, the Roy adaptation model, modeling and role modeling, Watson's theory of human caring, theories based on energy fields, the science of the unitary person, the theory of health as expanding consciousness, and the theory of human becoming.

**Theory into Practice:** Analyze the interpretation of the case of Mr. S. according to selected theories (Exhibit 4–1). Explore the nursing interventions most consistent with specific nursing theories (Table 4–2).

## EXPERIENTIAL EXERCISES

(2 hours. Incorporation of sharing circles and experiential exercises is encouraged for class presentation.)

Have each student choose a nursing theory (Exhibit 4–1) and become familiar with the definition of that theory. Have students compare the ideas and concepts common to all nursing theories. Describe a clinical situation and have the student explore how the chosen nursing theory served as a guide in application of both the art and science of nursing in this situation. Integrate in this clinical situation specific elements of the theory that were used: nursing knowledge, nursing theory, expertise, intuition, and creativity. Reinforce the importance of using nursing theory to guide practice, education, and research.

## DIRECTIONS FOR FUTURE RESEARCH

Have students choose one or more research questions as an area to explore; students should review the literature, identify research findings that could be utilized in practice, and/or postulate additional research questions or hypotheses. Consult with a nurse researcher to help develop a research study. Encourage students to begin collecting articles that can support further investigation.

## NURSE HEALER REFLECTIONS

Encourage students to use the chapter reflective questions as a guide to journal entries for exploring, understanding, and validating presence and healing.

Chapter 5

# Holistic Ethics

## CHAPTER OBJECTIVES

Refer to chapter for specific theoretical, clinical, and personal objectives. These will provide guidelines for the integration of objectives in class presentation, experiential sessions, and student homework assignments.

## CHAPTER OVERVIEW

Holistic ethics provides the framework and guidelines for the development of a healing attitude and morality in healers. Ethics serves as a foundation to teach individuals specific strategies to release the self (ego) and to access the wisdom of the transpersonal dimension.

## PROCESS EXERCISE NO. 5

(15-minute opening experiential session using music and healing objects if desired.)

### Vision of Healing: Ethics in Our Changing World

As we explore our own moral values and behaviors, we are able to access events that help shape who we are and why we behave as we do. Then, as we link our personal behaviors with our daily life experiences, we move toward a deeper understanding of holism. As you guide students, ask them to reflect on the choices they make in different scenarios and to consider how their choices reflect their ethics.

Begin with a guided relaxation exercise (5 minutes) and gradually fade in music of choice. Suggest to students that they can close their eyes or leave their eyes open. Ask students who leave their eyes open to focus on a spot several feet in front of them. This allows for a greater ease in following the relaxation and imagery suggestions and reflective experience.

Using techniques for empowering relaxation and imagery scripts (see Chapters 21 and 22), gently weave into a guided imagery exercise the following reflective questions: What gives your life meaning and purpose? On what grounds do you base your routine decisions? your major life decisions? With what actions do you feel a deep sense of interconnection with yourself, with others, or with the universe? Add three to five more reflective questions about ethics from a holistic perspective. Bring closure to the imagery process.

With soft music still playing, invite students to record in a personal journal (3 to 5 minutes) any images, process questions and answers, or insight gained. Ask students to bring personal closure to this process. Gradually fade music out. Engage students in a gentle stretching exercise before the theory session begins.

## KEY CONCEPTS: THEORY AND RESEARCH

(1-hour presentation)

**OPTIONAL: GUEST SPEAKER(S) AND VIDEO(S)**

**Guest Speaker(s):** Invite one or more nurses experienced in ethical issues. Provide guest speaker(s) with the Instructor's Manual suggestions so the speaker(s) can become familiar with the students' assignment before class.

**Video(s):** Show a video of an ethical issue (rent from local video store or media catalogue or purchase for school video library). Following the video presentation, ask students for their reactions and comments. Discuss the video and answer questions.

**Definitions:** Review definitions and incorporate into presentation.

**The Nature of Ethical Problems:** Increase the students' awareness of the range and scope of ethical dilemmas. Introduce aspects of life-prolonging technology to illustrate the complexity of issues of death and dying.

**Morals and Principles:** Discuss the three primary principles of biomedical ethics. Introduce the four conditions of the principle of double effect. Discuss the meaning of these four conditions and integrate clinical examples.

**Traditional Ethical Theories:** Review the basic theories on which Western ethics is based. Introduce and discuss the terms *deontologic* and *teleologic* and define the meaning of each term. Integrate the presuppositions of the new theory of holistic ethics. Discuss the Code of Ethics for Holistic Nurses (Exhibit 5–1).

**Development of Holistic Ethics:** Discuss the underlying concept of the unity and integral wholeness of all people and of all nature that is identified and pursued by finding unity and wholeness within the self and within humanity.

**Holistic Ethics and Consciousness:** Discuss the concept and dimensions of consciousness. Explore the three levels of consciousness. Begin a discussion of how the levels of consciousness relate to the theory of holistic ethics.

**Analysis of Ethical Dilemmas:** Introduce the four-step concept of ethical analysis. Explore each of the four steps and relate each step to one or more clinical situations.

## EXPERIENTIAL EXERCISES

(2 hours. Incorporation of sharing circles and experiential exercises is encouraged for class presentation.)

**Case Analysis:** Present a case history/story, either from your own clinical experience or from the literature. Ask the students to refer to Jonsen's four-component analysis technique and then analyze the case history/story. Depending on the time available and the number of students present, you may include the following: holding small group discussions; writing the four components on a board, poster, or overhead projection and leading a class discussion of each component; or asking student group leaders to present their groups' analyses to the class.

Have students also discuss case studies from their personal life experiences. Encourage students to share other patient stories and to focus on the meaning of the symptoms, disease, illness, and use of specific symbols and metaphors.

**Advance Medical Directives:** Review the key points of the 1991 Patient Self-Determination Act. Discuss the assessment questions a nurse may consider asking during the intake interview.

**Storytelling:** Use the metaphor of storytelling to make points about ethical situations. Collect stories from the literature or share stories based on your own clinical experiences.

## DIRECTIONS FOR FUTURE RESEARCH

Have students choose one or more research questions as an area to explore; students should review the literature, identify research findings that could be utilized in practice, and/or postulate additional research questions or hypotheses. Consult with a nurse researcher to help develop a research study. Encourage students to begin collecting articles that can support further investigation.

## NURSE HEALER REFLECTIONS

Encourage students to use the chapter reflective questions as a guide to journal entries for exploring, understanding, and validating presence and healing.

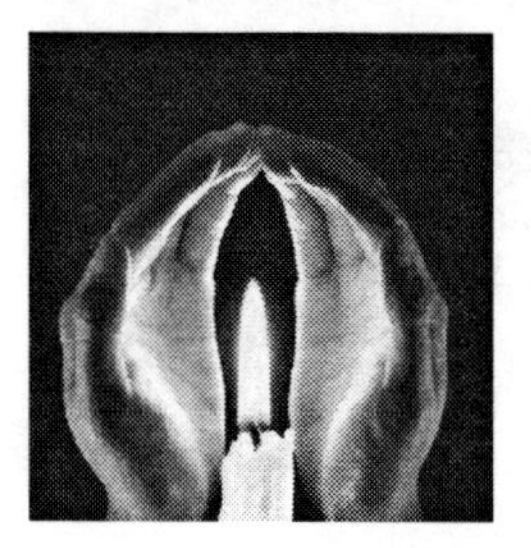

# CORE VALUE 2

# Holistic Education and Research

## Chapter 6

# The Psychophysiology of Bodymind Healing

### CHAPTER OBJECTIVES

Refer to chapter for specific theoretical, clinical, and personal objectives. These will provide guidelines for the integration of objectives in class presentation, experiential sessions, and student homework assignments.

### CHAPTER OVERVIEW

This chapter explores new developments in science that prompt us to view human beings in a new light. The mechanistic view of the world of Descartes and Newton is giving way to a holistic and ecologic view. Our habit of looking at individuals from the perspective of the body, mind, or spirit is misleading and creates problems of its own. New scientific understanding of living systems, such as principles of self-organization and Bell's theorem and mind modulation of the bodymind systems, provide a theoretical base for holistic healing interventions. Understanding of the physiologic principles involved in nursing interventions helps nurses to design individualized and appropriate holistic care for clients. Nurses, aware of their own personal woundedness and sensitive to the wounds of clients, are strategically placed to lead clients toward health and healing.

### PROCESS EXERCISE NO. 6

(15-minute opening experiential session using music and healing objects if desired.)

#### Vision of Healing: The Web of Life

Begin with a guided relaxation exercise (5 minutes) and gradually fade in music of choice. Suggest to students that they can close their eyes or leave their eyes open. Ask students who leave their eyes open to focus on a spot several feet in front of them. This allows for a greater ease in following the relaxation and imagery suggestions and reflective experience.

Using techniques for empowering relaxation and imagery scripts (see Chapters 21 and 22), gently weave into a guided imagery exercise the following reflection. Call up the image of a beautiful web of life and the interconnectedness of all parts of life, living and nonliving. Suggest that students incorporate all of the parts that make us whole—physical, mental, emotional, social, and spiritual. Invite students to add to their web of life all of those people, things, and places that help them in their healing journey. Invite them to recognize the parts of themselves that are wounded and the parts that need healing. Suggest that increased awareness of their strengths and the beautiful parts within their healing web can assist them in their lifelong journey into wholeness.

With soft music still playing, invite students to record in a personal journal (3 to 5 minutes) any images, process questions and answers, or insight gained. Ask students to bring personal closure to this process. Gradually fade music out. Engage students in a gentle stretching exercise before the theory session begins.

## KEY CONCEPTS: THEORY AND RESEARCH

(1-hour presentation)

**OPTIONAL: GUEST SPEAKER(S) AND VIDEO(S)**

**Guest Speaker(s):** Invite one or more nurses who use hypnotherapy in clinical practice to present the theory and to demonstrate different strategies for accessing state-dependent learning and memory. Provide guest speaker(s) with the Instructor's Manual suggestions so the speaker(s) can become familiar with students' assignment before class.

**Video(s):** Show a video that explores bodymind theories and modalities (rent from media catalogue or purchase for school video library). Following the video presentation, ask students for their reactions and comments. Discuss the video and answer questions.

**Definitions:** Review definitions and incorporate into presentation.

**Quantum Theory:** Review the major concepts in quantum theory and their importance to holistic nursing, health, and healing.

**Systems Theory:** Discuss concepts of human beings as living, open systems embedded in the web of life.

**Theory of Relativity:** Explore the idea contained in this theory that no absolute frame of reference exists independent of the observer. Apply this concept to holistic nursing, health, and healing.

**Principles of Self-Organization:** Discuss the principles of living organisms and nonliving things and explain the difference between them. Explore the ideas of internal, nonlinear feedback loops that are capable of self-organization.

**Bell's Theorem:** Discuss the dynamics of space and time as explained by Bell's theorem and the implications for health and healing.

**Personality and Wellness:** Discuss the relationship of personality characteristics to states of wellness.

**Information Theory:** Discuss how information theory is a mathematical model that emerged with modern communication technologies. Explain how information theory can unify physiologic, sociologic, and spiritual phenomenon and explain the connections between consciousness and bodymind healing.

**Santiago Theory of Cognition:** Explore how cognition and the transduction of information involves the whole process of life, including perception, emotions, and behavior.

**Emotions and the Neural Tripwire:** Discuss new information on transduction with the discovery of a small bundle of neurons that leads directly from the thalamus to the amygdala in addition to those that connect the neurocortex (Figure 6–1).

**State-Dependent Memory and Health:** Explore how state-dependent learning and memory influence how we perform and what we remember. Discuss the four integrated hypotheses regarding memory and learning. Connect this discussion with the opening process exercise.

**Location of Brain Centers:** Discuss the conflicts between the traditional neuroanatomic model, information theory, and mind modulation.

**Ultradian Rhythms:** Discuss the various natural biologic rhythms. Explore ultradian rhythms (Figure 6–2).

**Mind Modulation:** Explore mind modulation of all the body systems, keeping in mind that these systems act as a whole or in unison.

**Nervous System:** Discuss the nervous system and review Table 6–1 on sympathetic and parasympathetic responses to stress. Discuss the healing outcomes with regard to various body parts and body cells achievable with holistic modalities.

**Endocrine System:** Discuss the central tenet of neuroendocrinology—neurosecretion and its relationship to learning, memory, pain, perception, addictions, appetite, and so on. Examine hormones that have been identified as having bodymind function.

**Immune System:** Discuss the immune system and the bidirectional circuitry of these three systems. Examine the research discussed on the direct correlation between relaxation, imagery, and immunology.

**Neuropeptide System:** Discuss neuropeptides and their receptor sites, the bodymind interconnections, and the ways in which people experience emotions in their body.

**Pain Response:** Discuss the difference between acute pain and chronic pain.

**Psychosocial Pain Pathways:** Explore the cognitive and affective factors that influence pain. Give clinical examples to explain the interrelationship of physical pain and psychologic factors in the pain experience.

## EXPERIENTIAL EXERCISES

(2 hours. Incorporation of sharing circles and experiential exercises is encouraged for class presentation.)

**Clinical Implications for the Future:** Discuss the rapid changes in the knowledge of the psychophysiology of bodymind healing. Explore the challenges nurses face in clinical practice to refine the processes and techniques for specific modulation of bodymind symptoms. Integrate clinical examples.

Examine ultradian rhythms, ultradian stress syndrome, and ultradian performance rhythms. Review the major implications to consider in regard to the ultradian healing response (Figure 6–2).

Ask students to plot out the current day and to see at what times they have applied ultradian theory and healing strategies in their personal lives. What kept them from taking breaks, eating a nutritious lunch, exercising, and so on?

Have students integrate ultradian rhythms with one or more of their desired behavioral changes.

Encourage students to create a healing room for themselves at home. Ask students to explore with colleagues in the work environment ideas of ultradian breaks.

## DIRECTIONS FOR FUTURE RESEARCH

Have students choose one or more research questions as an area to explore; students should review the literature, identify research findings that could be utilized in practice, and/or postulate additional research questions or hypotheses. Consult with a nurse researcher to help develop a research study. Encourage students to begin collecting articles that can support further investigation.

## NURSE HEALER REFLECTIONS

Encourage students to use the chapter reflective questions as a guide to journal entries for exploring, understanding, and validating presence and healing.

# Chapter 7

# Spirituality and Health

## CHAPTER OBJECTIVES

Refer to chapter for specific theoretical, clinical, and personal objectives. These will provide guidelines for the integration of objectives in class presentation, experiential sessions, and student homework assignments.

## CHAPTER OVERVIEW

Spirituality is perhaps the most basic yet most misunderstood aspect of holistic nursing. Spirituality is the essence of who we are and how we are in the world and, like breathing, is essential to our human experience. Attending to spirituality across the lifespan implies an understanding of developmental aspects of spirituality and, in particular, recognition that awareness of and ways of expressing spirituality may vary with age. Spiritual caregiving requires an understanding that spirituality is broader than religion and a recognition that, although some people may not be religious, everyone is spiritual.

## PROCESS EXERCISE NO. 7

(15-minute opening experiential session using music and healing objects if desired.)

### Vision of Healing: The Evolving Process of Life's Dance

Healing ourselves and facilitating healing in others requires that we acknowledge the parts of our lives that need healing. The following exercise is an excellent example of state-dependent learning and memory (see Chapter 6). It demonstrates how to access a hurt from the past and how to reframe it to heal the hurt.

Share with students that the first part of this exercise is to remember a part of self that needs healing. The second part of the exercise is to create the healing. This process may bring tears, and different emotions may surface. If any students are uncomfortable with a memory that has been accessed, they can stay with the image and see what follows, or they can take a deep breath and open their eyes, and the images at that discomfort level will leave. There is no right or wrong way. If students choose not to participate at a deep level, suggest that they can intellectually perform the exercise and learn a tool for facilitating deep healing.

Begin with a guided relaxation exercise (5 minutes) and gradually fade in soft music of choice. Suggest to students that they can close their eyes or leave their eyes open. Ask students who leave their eyes open to focus on a spot several feet in front of them. This allows for a greater ease in following the relaxation and imagery suggestions and reflective experience.

Using techniques for empowering relaxation and imagery scripts (see Chapters 21 and 22), gently weave into a guided imagery exercise the following reflective questions.

Let yourself go back in time to between the ages of five and ten. If it seems right, allow a painful memory, a disappointment, or a failure to come into conscious awareness along with any details that may be remembered. Use all of your senses. Just be present and experience what comes into your awareness. It might be a time of remembering being embarrassed, feeling ashamed, or being physically or emotionally hurt. How old are you? What are you wearing? Where are you? Who is there with you? Stay with this experience for a while.

Now let yourself, in your wise grown-up voice, tell this little person that he or she is okay. With your loving-kindness, your compassion, tell this child comforting words that can bring about some healing of this experience. Hug or kiss the child. Just listen to the words, images, or feelings that come. You will know exactly what needs to be healed at this time. Tell the child within that you are always there and that you are always available to listen to past memories that are in need of healing. Next tell yourself that you are okay. Give yourself some thoughts about this part of yourself that still needs healing. Bring closure to the imagery process.

With soft music still playing, invite students to record in a personal journal (3 to 5 minutes) any images, process questions and answers, or insight gained. Ask students to bring personal closure to this process. Gradually fade music out. Engage students in a gentle stretching exercise before the theory session begins.

## KEY CONCEPTS: THEORY AND RESEARCH

(1-hour presentation)

**OPTIONAL: GUEST SPEAKER(S) AND VIDEO(S)**

**Guest Speaker(s):** Invite a nurse who integrates holistic modalities in clinical practice or a panel of nurses in different practice settings that are guided in practice by a bio-psycho-social-spiritual model. Provide guest speaker(s) with the Instructor's Manual suggestions so the speaker(s) can become familiar with the students' assignment before class.

**Video(s):** Show a video of a practitioner describing and demonstrating one or more holistic modalities (rent from media catalogue or purchase for school video library). Following the video presentation, ask students for their reactions and comments. Discuss the video and answer questions.

**Definitions:** Review definitions and incorporate into presentation.

**Relationship between Spirituality and Religion:** Define spirituality and religion and discuss the importance of each person's defining these two areas for his or her own life.

**Understanding Spirituality:** Explore the barriers and cultural definitions that are encountered regarding spirituality in nursing practice and personal life.

**Elements of Spirituality:** Explore the common elements in spirituality.

**Connectedness with the Sacred Source, Nature, Others, and Self:** Discuss how a person may experience a connectedness with the Sacred Source and the different names used to express the Sacred Source.

**Spirituality and the Healing Process:** Explore how mystery, love, suffering, hope, forgiveness, peace and peacemaking, grace, and prayer are inherent in the spiritual domain.

**Spirituality and Psychologic Dimensions:** Discuss the importance of recognizing the difference between the spiritual and the psychologic domains.

**Spirituality in Holistic Nursing:** Examine ways to dwell with, ponder, and incorporate unfolding spirituality into one's own life: ways to nurture the spirit, assessment and investigation of spirituality in practice and research, intentional listening and presence, story and metaphor in spiritual care, use of guides and instruments to facilitate spirituality assessment, tending to the spirit in holistic nursing practice, touch, fostering of connectedness, rituals to nurture the spirit, centering, mindfulness and awareness, prayer and meditation, rest and leisure, arts and spirituality.

## EXPERIENTIAL EXERCISES

(2 hours. Incorporation of sharing circles and experiential exercises is encouraged for class presentation.)

**Relationship between Spirituality and Religion:** Have students discuss the importance of each person's defining spirituality and religion in his or her own way. Ask students to share with each other their own personal definitions.

**Understanding Spirituality:** Have students explore the barriers and cultural definitions that are encountered regarding spirituality in nursing practice and personal life.

**Elements of Spirituality:** Ask students to share their personal definitions of spirituality. As these are being discussed, have one person write on a board the elements expressed by the group to further explore the concept of spirituality.

**Connectedness with the Sacred Source, Nature, Others, and Self:** Have students share their personal ways of experiencing connectedness with the Sacred Source.

**Spirituality and the Healing Process:** Have students share clinical or personal examples of mystery, love, suffering, hope, forgiveness, peace and peacemaking, grace, and prayer to further expand awareness of the spiritual domain.

**Spirituality and Psychologic Dimensions:** Have students share clinical or personal stories that illustrate the difference between the spiritual and the psychologic domains.

**Listening in Healing Ways:** Have students explore how to listen in healing ways (Exhibit 7–1).

**Facilitation of Awareness of Story:** Have students review ways to facilitate awareness of story (Exhibit 7–2). Provide time for personal sharing using any of these special ways to enhance one's story.

**Characteristics of Spirituality:** Have students work in dyads and take turns asking questions from the Spiritual Assessment Tool (Exhibit 7–3) categories of *meaning* and *purpose, inner strengths,* and *interconnections.* Assess those questions that are easy to answer and those that are difficult. Explore Howden's Spirituality Assessment Scale (Exhibit 7-4) and Barker's Spiritual Well-Being Assessment Instruments (Exhibit 7–5).

Invite students to share with the group their insights and experiences in evoking personal information in the three areas listed above. Have students explore the differences in answering these questions intellectually and being guided in an imagery exercise using these questions as in process exercise no. 1 at the beginning of an earlier class. Repeat a guided imagery exercise using the questions from the Spiritual Assessment Tool.

## DIRECTIONS FOR FUTURE RESEARCH

Have students choose one or more research questions as an area to explore; students should review the literature, identify research findings that could be utilized in practice, and/or postulate additional research questions or hypotheses. Consult with a nurse researcher to help develop a research study. Encourage students to begin collecting articles that can support further investigation.

## NURSE HEALER REFLECTIONS

Encourage students to use the chapter reflective questions as a guide to journal entries for exploring, understanding, and validating presence and healing.

# Chapter 8

# Energetic Healing

## CHAPTER OBJECTIVES

Refer to chapter for specific theoretical, clinical, and personal objectives. These will provide guidelines for the integration of objectives in class presentation, experiential sessions, and student homework assignments.

## CHAPTER OVERVIEW

Energetic healing is a concept based on theories from the fields of energy medicine and subtle energy. Energetic medicine includes all energetic informational interactions resulting from self-regulation or brought about through other energy couplings to mind and body. Subtle energies are said to move in the etheric body and are difficult to measure at present. Energetic healing is examined from historical and cutting-edge perspectives.

## PROCESS EXERCISE NO. 8

(15-minute opening experiential session using music and healing objects if desired.)

### Vision of Healing: Toward Wholeness

The practitioner of energetic healing has a knowledge of both scientific and conceptual theories. Skill and focused attention are directed to subtle and nonphysical aspects of the bodymind. A knowledgeable practitioner has undertaken his or her own healing journey in the process of self-development.

Begin with a guided relaxation exercise (5 minutes) and gradually fade in music of choice. Suggest to students that they can close their eyes or leave their eyes open. Ask students who leave their eyes open to focus on a spot several feet in front of them. This allows for a greater ease in following the relaxation and imagery suggestions and reflective experience.

Using techniques and empowering relaxation and imagery scripts (see Chapters 21 and 22), gently weave reflective questions into a guided imagery exercise and ask students to remember an event or time at which spontaneous hilarity was present. Encourage them to engage in the moment, remembering as many details as possible and using all of their senses. Invite them to laugh out loud as they evoke this special memory. Bring closure to the imagery process.

With soft music still playing, invite students to record in a personal journal (3 to 5 minutes) any images, process questions and answers, or insight gained. Ask students to bring personal closure to this process. Gradually fade music out. Engage students in a gentle stretching exercise before the theory session begins.

## KEY CONCEPTS: THEORY AND RESEARCH

(1-hour presentation)

**OPTIONAL: GUEST SPEAKER(S) AND VIDEO(S)**

**Guest Speaker(s):** Invite a nurse and/or clown experienced in play and laughter therapies. Provide guest speaker(s) with the Instructor's Manual suggestions so the speaker(s) can become familiar with the students' assignment before class.

**Video(s):** Show a video that evokes play and laughter (rent from local video store or media catalogue or purchase for school video library). Following the video presentation, ask students for their reactions and comments. Discuss the video and answer questions.

**Definitions:** Review definitions and incorporate into presentation.

**The Energetic Human:** Chakras and Aura Meridians: Discuss anatomy, traditions, and data on the 12 pairs of meridian pathways in the human body.

**Intuition:** Review the physiology of the neurotransmitter system and discuss how it relates to intuition.

**Chakras:** Review the chakra representations listed in Table 8–1. Examine Table 8–2 to identify how the chakras are associated with the nervous system or a neuroendocrine gland. Review Table 8–3 to discuss the theory of chronologic age and chakra development.

**Physics Metaphors:** Discuss how a chakra tree is like a Fourier analyzer or a spectrometer.

**The Aura:** The aura is traditionally described as a multilayer field of energy surrounding the physical body. Discuss several theorists' contributions to this area of thought. Examine Table 8–4 to guide the discussion.

**Holographic Theory:** Review and discuss holographic theory as it relates to physical beings. Give an example.

**Consciousness-Created Reality:** Review the quantum theory of how we may create energetic informational patterns and how we may heal them.

**Other Forms of Energy:** All the senses receive data. Discuss how these data are related to subtle energies.

## HOLISTIC CARING PROCESS

Focus on specifics of assessment, patterns/challenges/needs, outcomes, therapeutic care plan, implementation, and evaluation. Instruct students in the importance of developing their own style of preparation before, at the beginning of, during, and at the end of the session.

## EXPERIENTIAL EXERCISES

(2 hours. Incorporation of sharing circles and experiential exercises is encouraged in class presentation.)

**Awareness:** Direct students to spend some time in focused concentration to increase awareness of non-physical dimensions. Have students write down their perceptions.

**Intuition:** Have students work in dyads to practice developing intuitive skills. Direct students to practice this skill in their hours away from the classroom.

## DIRECTIONS FOR FUTURE RESEARCH

Have students choose one or more research questions as an area to explore; students should review the literature, identify research findings that could be utilized in practice, and/or postulate additional research questions or hypotheses. Consult with a nurse researcher to develop a research study. Encourage students to begin collecting articles that can support further investigation.

## NURSE HEALER REFLECTIONS

Encourage students to use the chapter reflective questions as a guide to journal entries for exploring, understanding, and validating presence and healing.

# Chapter 9

# Holistic Nursing Research

## CHAPTER OBJECTIVES

Refer to chapter for specific theoretical, clinical, and personal objectives. These will provide guidelines for the integration of objectives in class presentation, experiential sessions, and student homework assignments.

## CHAPTER OVERVIEW

A significant body of research provides evidence of the enormous effects of consciousness on both health and illness. Investigators have shown that complementary and alternative therapies have the exciting potential to prevent illness and maintain high-level wellness. Such research has been instrumental in guiding the development of humanistic and holistic health care. The challenge for nursing is to apply these findings in nursing practice.

## PROCESS EXERCISE NO. 9

(15-minute opening experiential session using music and healing objects if desired.)

### Vision of Healing: Questioning the Rules of Science

Nurses have traditionally relied on accumulated practical experience as though it were equivalent to knowledge. Nothing is more effective in shaking loose this belief than a confrontation with the fact that not everyone's experience leads to the same conclusion. It is when we explore new concepts and possibilities that we make breakthroughs into new clinical practice possibilities to improve the quality of care.

Begin with a guided relaxation exercise (5 minutes) and gradually fade in music of choice. Suggest to students that they can close their eyes or leave their eyes open. Ask students who leave their eyes open to focus on a spot several feet in front of them. This allows for a greater ease in following the relaxation and imagery suggestions and reflective experience.

Using techniques for empowering relaxation and imagery scripts (see Chapters 21 and 22), gently weave into a guided imagery exercise reflective questions such as the following: How do I utilize research findings to guide my clinical practice? Do I find opportunities to incorporate the results of research to update the principal interventions I use in my practice? Do I have opportunities but fail to take advantage of them? Is there a research problem or interest area that I would like to explore? Add three to five more reflective questions about research. Bring closure to the imagery process.

With soft music still playing, invite students to record in a personal journal (3 to 5 minutes) any images, process questions and answers, or insight gained. Ask students to bring personal closure to this process. Gradually fade music out. Engage students in a gentle stretching exercise before the theory session begins.

## KEY CONCEPTS: THEORY AND RESEARCH

(1-hour presentation)
**OPTIONAL: GUEST SPEAKER(S) AND VIDEO(S)**

**Guest Speaker(s):** Invite one or more nurses experienced in clinical research. Provide guest speaker(s) with the Instructor's Manual suggestions so the speaker(s) can become familiar with the students' assignment before class.

**Video(s):** Show a video of a nurse researcher describing and demonstrating one or more aspects of clinical research (rent from media catalogue or purchase for school video library). Following the video presentation, ask students for their reactions and comments. Discuss the video and answer questions.

**Definitions:** Review definitions and incorporate into presentation.

**Wellness Model:** Discuss how the framework of client/patient nursing research is shifting from an illness to a wellness model of health care.

**Evidence-Based Practice:** Analyze why holistic care of clients/patients must be based on the best evidence to direct our clinical decisions and actions and why additional research in holistic nursing and complementary and alternative therapies is essential. Compare differences between the process of research utilization and evidence-based practice. Explore the resources available to help practitioners obtain information about evidence-based practice (e.g., research studies, practice guidelines developed by expert consensus and federal and professional groups, review articles, procedure manuals, and books) to update clinical policies, procedures, and standards of practice.

**Holistic Research Methods:** Review the four categories of quantitative research and the five types of qualitative research. Compare the purpose of quantitative research to that of qualitative research. Review the descriptive expressions of participants about the experience of health (Table 9–1). Compare and contrast qualitative and quantitative methodologies (Exhibits 9–1 and 9–2). Discuss how both methodologies are needed in holistic research.

**Enhancing Holistic Research:** Discuss various triangulation strategies to enhance the holistic nature of a research study. Explore the need for psychophysiologic measurement tools to evaluate holistic interventions. Discuss why multimodal interventions may have powerful affects on clinical outcomes. Review Heisenberg's Uncertainty Principle and its implications for holistic research. Examine the placebo response and its effects on clinical practice and research.

## EXPERIENTIAL EXERCISES

(2 hours. Incorporation of sharing circles and experiential exercises is encouraged for class presentation.)

**Holistic Measurement Tools:** Review several research tools that measure a client's physical, psychological, social, and spiritual dimensions.

**Multimodal Interventions:** Explore how various interventions might be combined into a multimodal intervention package to enhance outcomes.

**Draft of a Research Proposal:** Ask students to review the chapter section entitled "Directions for Future Research" as a guide for this exercise. Have students work in groups of three to five individuals over several weeks to draft a holistically oriented research proposal. Provide time for guidance, consultation, discussion, and critique of proposal drafts.

## DIRECTIONS FOR FUTURE RESEARCH

Have students choose one or more research questions as an area to explore; students should review the literature, identify research findings that could be utilized in practice, and/or postulate additional research questions or hypotheses. Consult with a nurse researcher to help develop a research study. Encourage students to begin collecting articles and clinical ideas that can support further investigation.

## NURSE HEALER REFLECTIONS

Encourage students to use chapter reflective questions as a guide to journal entries for exploring, understanding, and validating presence and healing.

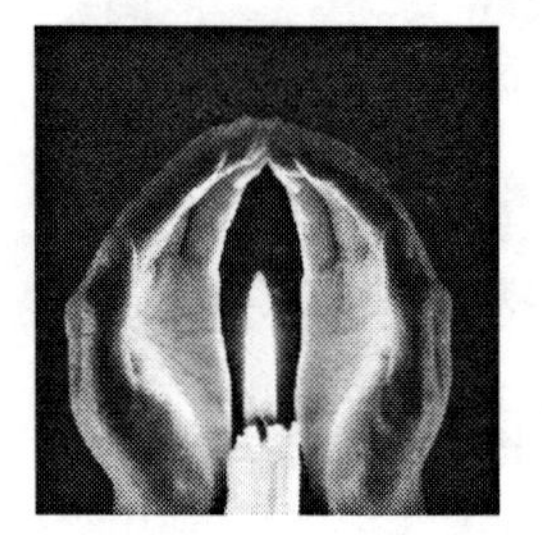

# CORE VALUE 3

## Holistic Nurse Self-Care

## Chapter 10

# The Nurse As an Instrument of Healing

### CHAPTER OBJECTIVES

Refer to chapter for specific theoretical, clinical, and personal objectives. These will provide guidelines for the integration of objectives in class presentation, experiential sessions, and student homework assignments.

### CHAPTER OVERVIEW

Awareness of being an instrument of healing allows the nurse an opportunity to explore the inner dimensions of personal, interpersonal, and transpersonal growth. Awareness of healing and being a healer allows a presence that gives new dimensions to the nurse's interactions with the client/patient.

### PROCESS EXERCISE NO. 10

(15-minute opening experiential session using music and healing objects if desired.)

#### Vision of Healing: Toward the Inward Journey

True nurse healing requires attention to one's strengths and weaknesses, and to purpose and meaning in life. As the parts of self that need healing are discovered, the nurse is able to be more fully present in the moment to assist others with their healing.

Begin with a guided relaxation exercise (5 minutes) and gradually fade in soft music of choice. Suggest to students that they can close their eyes or leave their eyes open. Ask students who leave their eyes open to focus on a spot several feet in front of them. This allows for a greater ease in following the relaxation and imagery suggestions and reflective experience.

Using techniques for empowering relaxation and imagery scripts (see Chapters 21 and 22), gently weave into a guided imagery exercise reflective questions related to the characteristics and qualities of a nurse healer. Suggest to students that they resonate with each characteristic and quality and notice which have a ring of truth and which need to be developed. Bring closure to the imagery process.

With soft music still playing, invite students to record in a personal journal (3 to 5 minutes) any images, process questions and answers, or insight gained. Ask students to bring personal closure to this process. Gradually fade music out. Engage students in a gentle stretching exercise before the theory session begins.

### KEY CONCEPTS: THEORY AND RESEARCH

(1-hour presentation)
OPTIONAL: GUEST SPEAKER(S) AND VIDEO(S)

**Guest Speaker(s):** Invite one or more nurses who are exploring the concept of presence and healing in clinical practice. Provide guest speaker(s) with the Instructor's Manual suggestions so the speaker(s) can become familiar with the students' assignment before class.

**Video(s):** Show a video of a nurse or nurses describing and demonstrating presence and healing in clinical practice (rent from media catalogue or purchase for school video library). Following the video presentation, ask students for their reactions and comments. Discuss the video and answer questions.

**Definitions:** Review definitions and incorporate into presentation.

**Concept of Healing:** Examine the concepts within healing and build on discussion from previous class.

**Presence:** Discuss the multidimensional state of presence: physical presence, psychologic presence, and therapeutic presence (Table 10–1).

**Nature of Healing Relationships:** Explore the nature, depth, and degree of connection and interaction between the self, other, creator, and creation.

**The Nurse As a Healing Environment:** Explore the qualities that the nurse can use to enhance healing and expand ideas from previous sessions.

**Healing Interventions, Outcomes, and Evaluation:** Discuss the process of preparing for healing interventions, identifying outcomes, and evaluating a healing intervention.

## EXPERIENTIAL EXERCISES

(2 hours. Incorporation of sharing circles and experiential exercises is encouraged for class presentation.)

**Presence:** Further explore the three levels of presence—physical, psychologic, and therapeutic—and the healing qualities and states in each level (Table 10–1). Have students give personal and clinical examples of each. Discuss how the art of guiding requires skills of presence. These skills can be developed in many ways, such as through mindfulness practice, relaxation, imagery, music, and so forth. Explore the importance of self-care to be present in one's work. Explore the journey of working and living from a holistic perspective.

## DIRECTIONS FOR FUTURE RESEARCH

Have students choose one or more research questions as an area to explore; students should review the literature, identify research findings that could be utilized in practice, and/or postulate additional research questions or hypotheses. Consult with a nurse researcher to help develop a research study. Encourage students to begin collecting articles that can support further investigation.

## NURSE HEALER REFLECTIONS

Encourage students to use chapter reflective questions as a guide to journal entries for exploring, understanding, and validating presence and healing.

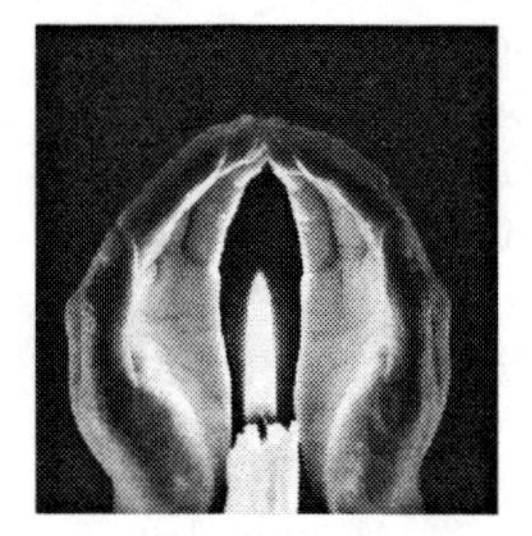

# CORE VALUE 4

# Holistic Communication, Therapeutic Environment, and Cultural Diversity

## Chapter 11

# Therapeutic Communication: The Art of Helping

### CHAPTER OBJECTIVES

Refer to chapter for specific theoretical, clinical, and personal objectives. These will provide guidelines for the integration of objectives in class presentation, experiential sessions, and student homework assignments.

### CHAPTER OVERVIEW

Therapeutic communication is a systematic way of relating to another person to enhance self-discovery. It builds a positive, supportive relationship from which the client can explore his or her personal experience and behavior. The helper must use many personal skills to achieve a focused interaction.

### PROCESS EXERCISE NO. 11

(15-minute opening experiential session using music and healing objects if desired.)

#### Vision of Healing: Human Care

The human care process between a nurse and another individual is a special, delicate gift to be cherished. The human care transactions make it possible for two individuals to come together and establish contact; one person's body-mind-spirit joins another's body-mind-spirit in a lived moment.

Begin with a guided relaxation exercise (5 minutes) and gradually fade in music of choice. Suggest to students that they can close their eyes or leave their eyes open. Ask students who leave their eyes open to focus on a spot several feet in front of them. This allows for a greater ease in following the relaxation and imagery suggestions and reflective experience.

Using techniques for empowering relaxation and imagery scripts (see Chapters 21 and 22), gently weave into a guided imagery exercise reflective questions about the ways in which the special shared moment of the present has the potential to transcend time, space, and the physical world. Invite students to bring into their imagery process special shared moments with clients. Bring closure to the imagery process.

With soft music still playing, invite students to record in a personal journal (3 to 5 minutes) any images, process questions and answers, or insight gained. Ask students to bring personal closure to this process. Gradually fade music out. Engage students in a gentle stretching exercise before the theory session begins.

## KEY CONCEPTS: THEORY AND RESEARCH

(1-hour presentation)

**OPTIONAL: GUEST SPEAKER(S) AND VIDEO(S)**

**Guest Speaker(s):** Invite one or more nurses who integrate therapeutic ocmmunication as a primary part of their practice. Provide guest speaker(s) with the Instructor's Manual suggestions so the speaker(s) can become familiar with the students' assignment before class.

**Video(s):** Show a video of a practitioner describing and demonstrating therapeutic communication with clients for self-discovery (rent from media catalogue or purchase for school video library). Following the video presentation, ask students for their reactions and comments. Discuss the video and answer questions.

**Definitions:** Review definitions and incorporate into presentation.

**Communication:** Examine the process of communication.

**Therapeutic Communication:** Discuss the helper's role in therapeutic communication.

**Therapeutic Communication Helping Model:** Explore the three stages of the therapeutic communication helping model.

**Therapeutic Communication Skills:** Examine the therapeutic communication skills that must be mastered within each of the three stages of the therapeutic communication helping model.

## EXPERIENTIAL EXERCISES

(2 hours. Incorporation of sharing circles and experiential exercises is encouraged for class presentation.)

**Empathic Responses:** Have students practice empathic responses that connect feelings and reasons for the feelings.

**Additive Empathic Responses:** Have students practice additive empathic responses with one another to uncover deeper or underlying feelings.

**Thematic Statements:** Have students practice thematic statements that include the triggering event or stimulus, the pattern of response, and the consequence of the behavior.

**Personalization of Additive Empathy:** Ask students to personalize additive empathy by practicing statements that include self-judgments, deficit behavior, and goal behavior.

**Feedback:** Have students practice feedback statements with one another.

**Confrontation:** Have students practice confrontation statements with one another to examine discrepancies in behavior.

**Immediacy:** Invite students to practice immediacy statements for exploring the here and now.

**Implementation:** Invite students to experience the skills of problem solving by clarifying goals, brainstorming options, selecting alternatives, formulating a specific action plan, and troubleshooting the plan.

## DIRECTIONS FOR FUTURE RESEARCH

Have students choose one or more research questions as an area to explore; students should review the literature, identify research findings that could be utilized in practice, and/or postulate additional research questions or hypotheses. Consult with a nurse researcher to help develop a research study. Encourage students to begin collecting articles that can support further investigation.

## NURSE HEALER REFLECTIONS

Encourage students to use the chapter reflective questions as a guide to journal entries for exploring, understanding, and validating presence and healing.

# Chapter 12

# Environment

## CHAPTER OBJECTIVES

Refer to chapter for specific theoretical, clinical, and personal objectives. These will provide guidelines for the integration of objectives in class presentation, experiential sessions, and student homework assignments.

## CHAPTER OVERVIEW

Environment and its many uses are among the foremost issues of the twenty-first century. Nurses are emerging as leaders in educating others about the benefit of working together to protect and enhance personal and community environmental spaces. The air we breathe, the sounds we hear, and the space we see all affect how we feel, think, and function.

## PROCESS EXERCISE NO. 12

(15-minute opening experiential session using music and healing objects if desired.)

### Vision of Healing: Building a Healthy Environment

"Every day we find a new sky and a new earth with which we are entrusted like a perfect toy. We are given the salty river of our blood winding through us, to remember the sea and our kindred under the waves."[1]

As we explore our personal environments, we become increasingly aware of the effects of our actions and behaviors on the whole planet. On an individual level, the way in which people use their personal space affects not only the way they feel but also, in today's shrinking world, the space within and around others.

Begin with a guided relaxation exercise (5 minutes) and gradually fade in music of choice. Suggest to students that they can close their eyes or leave their eyes open. Ask students who leave their eyes open to focus on a spot several feet in front of them. This allows for a greater ease in following the suggestions and reflective experience.

Using techniques for empowering relaxation and imagery scripts (see Chapters 21 and 22), gently weave into a guided imagery exercise reflective questions about the space in which students currently live and work. Have students reflect on the aesthetics, the aromas, the sounds, and the sights of their internal and external environments. Ask them to consider what a healing environment would be like. Bring closure to the imagery process.

With soft music still playing, invite students to record in a personal journal (3 to 5 minutes) any images, process questions and answers, or insight gained. Ask students to bring personal closure to this process. Gradually fade music out. Engage students in a gentle stretching exercise before the theory session begins.

## KEY CONCEPTS: THEORY AND RESEARCH

(1-hour presentation)
OPTIONAL: GUEST SPEAKER(S) AND VIDEO(S)

**Guest Speaker(s):** Invite one or more nurses experienced in environmental issues. Provide guest speaker(s) with the Instructor's Manual suggestions so the speaker(s) can become familiar with the students' assignment before class.

**Video(s):** Show a video about environmental issues (rent from local video store or media catalogue or purchase for school video library). Following the video presentation, ask students for their reactions and comments. Discuss the video and answer questions.

**Definitions:** Review definitions and incorporate into presentation.

**Theme One—Telling Our Story:** Discuss in groups what it means to be an earth citizen. Also explore the evolution of human consciousness and the core elements driving the multidimensional crisis of the planet.

**Theme Two—Living in a Toxic World:** Explore ways in which we can meet our needs on this planet without destroying our life-support systems. Examine three key principles that might be used as guidelines and policy for reducing pollution in the environment. Discuss four major categories of questions that can be asked when potential products are considered for use to lead to a less toxic world.

**Theme Three—Choosing a Sustainable Future:** Discuss principles and activities that will assist each of us to participate in creating a sustainable future.

**Theme Four—Building Learning Communities:** Explore the concept of learning communities that are characterized by safety, support, and openness, and discuss how such communities are fostering a just, sustainable, and compassionate future.

**Theme Five—Working from the Inside Out:** Discuss our day-to-day choices in life and work that can lead to environmental sustainability.

**The Modern Dilemma:** Review current environmental concerns (Figure 12–1). Discuss how they affect all earth dwellers. Ask for suggestions on how each individual can make a difference.

**American Holistic Nurses' Association Statement in Support of a Healthful Environment:** Discuss the stance of the American Holistic Nurses' Association regarding a healthful environment.

**Noise:** Explore how noise may be one of the most common environmental health hazards. Discuss the physiologic and psychologic effects of noise pollution and steps to help correct it.

**Food Irradiation:** Discuss both positive and negative effects of the controversial food irradiation program.

**Meat and Poultry Supplementation:** Have an open discussion on the pros and cons of meat and poultry supplementation.

**Smoking:** Engage students in discussion of situations in which the documented environmental smoking hazard affects them on a daily basis. Ask students to consider strategies to decrease this health hazard in their personal and work environments.

**Nurses' Work Environment:** Discuss a variety of health care delivery environments such as acute care, long-term care, and home health care. Encourage students to identify potential environmental hazards and possible ways to correct or avoid them.

## HOLISTIC CARING PROCESS

Focus on specifics of assessment, patterns/challenges/needs, outcomes, therapeutic care plan, implementation, and evaluation (Table 12–2 and Exhibit 12–2). Instruct students in the importance of developing their own style of preparation before, at the beginning of, during, and at the end of the session.

## EXPERIENTIAL EXERCISES

(2 hours. Incorporation of sharing circles and experiential exercises is encouraged for class presentation. Refer to the chapter section entitled "Specific Interventions" for details.)

**Personal Environment:** Engage students in a reflective experience of bringing to mind their personal living space and its healing aspects as well as those areas that are in need of healing. Have students briefly share their experiences and also share what was learned from sharing with others. In another guided imagery exercise, ask students to close their eyes and listen carefully to all the sounds in their current environment. Follow the steps suggested in the text for recording and analyzing what was heard.

**Workplace Hazards:** Discuss workplace hazards. Follow the suggested steps (Table 12–3) to identify possible problems and solutions.

**Planetary Consciousness:** Develop a guided imagery and music exercise with a central focus or theme of interconnectedness and of working together to enhance our planetary home. This exercise allows students to deepen their experience of creating their own special place in the universe and to identify how their individual actions work together to create the whole.

**Case Study:** Have students discuss case studies and incorporate a case study into group presentation. Encourage students to share other client/patient stories and to focus on the meaning of the symptoms, disease, illness, and use of specific symbols and metaphors.

### DIRECTIONS FOR FUTURE RESEARCH

Have students choose one or more research questions as an area to explore; students should review the literature, identify research findings that could be utilized in practice, and/or postulate additional research questions or hypotheses. Consult with a nurse researcher to help develop a research study. Encourage students to begin collecting articles that can support further investigation.

### NURSE HEALER REFLECTIONS

Encourage students to use the chapter reflective questions as a guide to journal entries for exploring, understanding, and validating presence and healing.

### NOTES

1. From *Available Light* by Marge Piercey, copyright © 1988 by Middlemarsh, Inc. and *The Art of Blessing the Day* by Marge Piercey, copyright © 1999 by Middlemarsh, Inc. Reprinted by permission of Alfred A. Knop, Inc. and the Wallace Literary Agency, Inc.

## Chapter 13

# Cultural Diversity and Care

### CHAPTER OBJECTIVES

Refer to chapter for specific theoretical, clinical, and personal objectives. These will provide guidelines for the integration of objectives in class presentation, experiential sessions, and student homework assignments.

### CHAPTER OVERVIEW

With global awareness of multiple cultures, cultural competency is increasingly important for nurses. Nurses working in culturally pluralistic societies must understand the history, values, and beliefs of other cultural groups as well as factors in migration. A key element in acquiring this competency is the twofold awareness of one's own cultural orientations and those of the client. Nurses must continue to develop cultural competency to provide holistic patient care.

### PROCESS EXERCISE NO. 13

(15-minute opening experiential session using music and healing objects if desired.)

#### Vision of Healing: Sharing Our Healing Stories

Do you have trouble talking about healing and what you do as a nurse to facilitate healing? Common comments by nurses are, "Well, that is what I do because I am a nurse," or "It is expected that I help patients." Frequently, nurses fail to give themselves credit for healing moments; this failure can lead to burnout and a feeling of "same old thing, day in and day out." When was the last time you created time within yourself to affirm the value of your actions and your presence with yourself or another? Can you recall saying to yourself, "I did a wonderful job," and then feeling inspired about your work and healing interactions?

Begin with a guided relaxation exercise (5 minutes) and gradually fade in music of choice. Suggest to students that they can close their eyes or leave their eyes open. Ask students who leave their eyes open to focus on a spot several feet in front of them. This allows for a greater ease in following the relaxation and imagery suggestions and reflective experience.

Using techniques for empowering relaxation and imagery (see Chapters 21 and 22), gently weave into a guided imagery exercise reflective questions such as the following: Can you remember a case in which your actions and your presence were important to another? Can you recall a client-nurse exchange in which you felt you did a wonderful job and were inspired about your work and healing interactions? Add three to five more reflective questions. Bring closure to the imagery process.

With soft music still playing, invite students to record in a personal journal (3 to 5 minutes) any images, process questions and answers, or insight gained. Ask students to bring personal closure to this process. Gradually fade music out. Engage students in a gentle stretching exercise before the theory session begins.

## KEY CONCEPTS: THEORY AND RESEARCH

(1-hour presentation)
**OPTIONAL: GUEST SPEAKER(S) AND VIDEO(S)**

**Guest Speaker(s):** Invite one or more nurses experienced in cultural diversity. Provide guest speaker(s) with the Instructor's Manual suggestions so the speaker(s) can become familiar with the students' assignment before class.

**Video(s):** Show a video of a nurse demonstrating one or more aspects of culturally competent care (rent from media catalogue or purchase for school video library). Following the video presentation, ask students for their reactions and comments. Discuss the video and answer questions.

**Definitions:** Review definitions and incorporate into presentation.

**Cultural Competency:** Explore the five components of culturally competent care.

**Cultural Diversity:** Discuss seven variables that influence cultural grouping.

**Common Myths and Errors Regarding Cultural Diversity:** Explore four common myths and errors related to cultural diversity.

**Factors That Affect the Development of Cultural Patterns and Behaviors:** Discuss the way in which geography, gender, value orientations, cultural beliefs, and technology contribute to cultural patterns and behaviors.

**Ethnic Groups in North America:** Compare and contrast the cultures of Native Americans, European Americans, African Americans, Asian Americans, Pacific Islanders and Native Hawaiians, and Hispanic or Latino Americans.

**Impact of Culture on Health Care:** Discuss the influence of cross-cultural paradigms, cultural sectors, and explanatory models on cultural understanding of health and illness.

**Nursing Applications for Developing Cultural Competency:** Explore the way in which communication and translators facilitate culturally competent care (Figure B–1).

## HOLISTIC CARING PROCESS

Focus on specifics of assessment, patterns/challenges/needs, outcomes, therapeutic care plan, implementation, and evaluation for culturally competent care. Instruct students in the importance of developing their own style of preparation before, at the beginning of, during, and at the end of the session.

## EXPERIENTIAL EXERCISES

(2 hours. Incorporation of sharing circles and experiential exercises is encouraged for class presentation.)

**Components of Transcultural Assessment:** Analyze the six components of a systematic transcultural client assessment and discuss techniques that can be used to obtain a cultural assessment.

**Modes of Cultural Intervention:** Have students explore the three modes of intervention involving clinical decision making that include the client's cultural practices and discuss a case study demonstrating how these modes can be incorporated into practice.

## DIRECTIONS FOR FUTURE RESEARCH

Have students choose one or more research questions as an area to explore; students should review the literature, identify research findings that could be utilized in practice, and/or postulate additional research questions or hypotheses. Consult with a nurse researcher to help develop a research study. Encourage students to begin collecting articles that can support further investigation.

## NURSE HEALER REFLECTIONS

Encourage students to use chapter reflective questions as a guide to journal entries for exploring, understanding, and validating presence and healing.

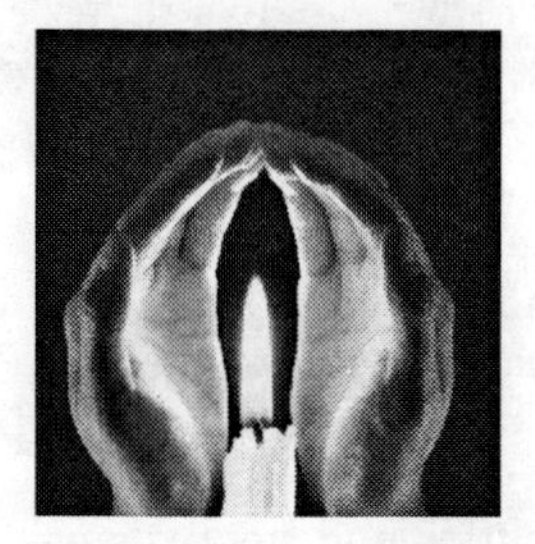

# CORE VALUE 5

## Holistic Caring Process

### Chapter 14

# The Holistic Caring Process

## CHAPTER OBJECTIVES

Refer to chapter for specific theoretical, clinical, and personal objectives. These will provide guidelines for the integration of objectives in class presentation, experiential sessions, and student homework assignments.

## CHAPTER OVERVIEW

The holistic caring process is an adaptation of the nursing process that incorporates holistic nursing philosophy and nursing theories. The holistic caring process is a systematic, dynamic living framework for discovering, describing, and documenting health patterns unique to the person. It is a six-step circular process involving assessment, patterns/problems/needs, outcomes, therapeutic care plan, implementation, and evaluation. The holistic caring process is contained in the American Holistic Nurses' Association (AHNA) Standards of Holistic Nursing Practice, which define and establish the scope of holistic nursing practice (Appendix 1-A).

## PROCESS EXERCISE NO. 14

(15-minute opening experiential session using music and healing objects if desired.)

### Vision of Healing: Working with Others

Human care involves a client-centered, focused process of caring and healing. As nurses explore holistic principles and develop the skills of self-care and presence, human care is at the core of all actions.

Begin with a guided relaxation exercise (5 minutes) and gradually fade in music of choice. Suggest to students that they can close their eyes or leave their eyes open. Ask students who leave their eyes open to focus on a spot several feet in front of them. This allows for a greater ease in following the relaxation and imagery suggestions and reflective experience.

Using techniques for empowering relaxation and imagery scripts (see Chapters 21 and 22), gently weave into a guided imagery exercise reflective questions that use the nursing process framework. In the imagination, slowly guide students in assessing and diagnosing their own body-mind-spirit. Then ask them to create an outcome, plan, and intervention for achieving more balance and harmony in one area of their lives. Finally, ask them to imagine an evaluation process for the desired outcome. Bring closure to the imagery process.

With soft music still playing, invite students to record in a personal journal (3 to 5 minutes) any images, process questions and answers, or insight gained. Ask students to bring personal closure to this process. Gradually fade music out. Engage students in a gentle stretching exercise before the theory session begins.

## KEY CONCEPTS: THEORY AND RESEARCH

(1-hour presentation)
**OPTIONAL: GUEST SPEAKER(S) AND VIDEO(S)**

**Guest Speaker(s):** Invite one or more nurses to discuss the dynamics of using and integrating a holistic assessment tool in clinical practice. Provide guest speaker(s) with the Instructor's Manual suggestions so the speaker(s) can become familiar with the students' assignment before class.

**Video(s):** Show a video of a practitioner who describes, demonstrates, and integrates holistic assessment tools and nursing process in clinical practice (rent from local video store or media catalogue or purchase for school video library). following the video presentation, ask students for their reactions and comments. Discuss the video and answer questions.

**Definitions:** Review definitions and incorporate into presentation.

## HOLISTIC CARING PROCESS

Focus on specifics of holistic assessment and intuitive thinking, patterns/challenges/needs (Exhibit 14-2, 14-3, and 14-4), outcomes, therapeutic care plans, implementation, and evaluation. Review the AHNA's 2003 Standards of Holistic Nursing Practice (Appendix 1-A).

## EXPERIENTIAL EXERCISES

(2 hours. Incorporation of caring circles and experiential exercises is encouraged in class presentation.)

**Holistic Assessment Tools:** Have students compare current assessment tools from different clinical settings to determine whether such tools focus on a holistic assessment. Explore the importance of using a holistic assessment tool and the ways in which a holistic assessment tool can help identify the client's patterns/challenges/needs more completely than a medical model systems assessment or a head-to-toe assessment tool with psychosocial questions added. Explore intuition and creativity as important aspects of a holistic assessment. Give examples from clinical and personal practice.

**Holistic Caring Process:** Engage students in dynamics of the holistic caring process through presentation of case studies involving holistic assessment, intuitive thinking, patterns/challenges/needs identification using the 13 domains of Taxonomy II and nursing diagnoses, outcomes, therapeutic care planning, implementation, and evaluation. Integrate the holistic caring process discussion with the AHNA Standards of Holistic Nursing Practice.

## DIRECTIONS FOR FUTURE RESEARCH

Have students choose one or more research questions as an area to explore; students should review the literature, identify research findings that could be utilized in practice, and/or postulate additional resaerch questions or hypotheses. Consult with a nurse researcher to help develop a research study. Encourage students to begin collecting articles that can support further investigation.

## NURSE HEALER REFLECTIONS

Encourage students to use the chapter reflective questions as a guide to journal entries for exploring, understanding, and validating presence and healing.

## Chapter 15

# Self-Assessments: Facilitating Healing in Self and Others

## CHAPTER OBJECTIVES

Refer to chapter for specific theoretical, clinical, and personal objectives. These will provide guidelines for the integration of objectives in class presentation, experiential sessions, and student homework assignments.

## CHAPTER OVERVIEW

Each of our human potentials affects our whole being. When we strive to develop all areas, a deeper sense of wholeness emerges, our self-worth increases, and life goals are actualized. Being alive becomes more exciting, rewarding, and fulfilling. Even when frustrations arise, individuals who assess their human potentials can more easily recognize and make effective choices and decrease the barriers to maximizing human potentials.

## PROCESS EXERCISE NO. 15

(15-minute opening experiential session using music and healing objects if desired)

### Vision of Healing: Actualization of Human Potentials

Our challenge in all aspects of our personal and professional lives is to strive to integrate all our human potentials. When we assess our human potentials and decide how we want our lives to be, we evoke meaning and purpose in life. If one area of our human potential is left undeveloped, life events do not seem as good as they could be.

Begin with a guided relaxation exercise (5 minutes) and gradually fade in music of choice. Suggest to students that they can close their eyes or leave their eyes open. Ask students who leave their eyes open to focus on a spot several feet in front of them. This allows for a greater ease in following the relaxation and imagery suggestions and reflective experience.

Using techniques for empowering relaxation and imagery scripts (see Chapters 21 and 22), gently weave into a guided imagery exercise reflective questions from each category of the human potential self-assessment. Imagine that you have a short period of time to share a healing moment and a hurting moment with someone who loves you. Invite into your imagination a person who loves you unconditionally who is available to you to listen actively. How important is this to the healing process? What steps would you take to begin this process? Bring closure to the imagery process.

With soft music still playing, invite students to record in a personal journal (3 to 5 minutes) any images, process questions and answers, or insight gained. Ask students to bring personal closure to this process. Gradually fade music out. Engage students in a gentle stretching exercise before the theory session begins.

## KEY CONCEPTS: THEORY AND RESEARCH

(1-hour presentation)

**Definitions:** Review definitions and incorporate into presentation.

**Circle of Human Potentials:** Examine the concept of body-mind-spirit as a complex feedback loop that is in a constant state of change. Explore each dimension of human potential—physical, mental, emotions, relationships, choices, and spirit (Figure 15–1).

## EXPERIENTIAL EXERCISES

(2 hours. Incorporation of sharing circles and experiential exercises is encouraged for class presentation.)

**Self-Assessments:** Explore the importance of self-assessment as a means of developing health and clarity of purpose and meaning in life. Have students complete the self-assessments (Figures 15–2 to 15–7) and tabulate scores (Exhibit 15–1). Allow time for students to work in dyads and to share areas that are the most challenging.

**Affirmations:** Guide students in an imagery exercise using several affirmations from each area of human potential (see boxes). Allow time for students to share experiences of affirming intentions and choices. Have students explore how affirmations can be of help in recognizing negative affirmations or changing a perception, attitude, belief, or value.

## DIRECTIONS FOR FUTURE RESEARCH

Have students choose one or more research questions as an area to explore; students should review the literature, identify research findings that could be utilized in practice, and/or postulate additional research questions or hypotheses. Consult with a nurse researcher to help develop a research study. Encourage students to begin collecting articles that can support further investigation.

## NURSE HEALER REFLECTIONS

Encourage students to use chapter reflective questions as a guide to journal entries for exploring, understanding, and validating presence and healing.

# Chapter 16

# Cognitive Therapy

## CHAPTER OBJECTIVES

Refer to chapter for specific theoretical, clinical, and personal objectives. These will provide guidelines for the integration of objectives in class presentation, experiential sessions, and student homework assignments.

## CHAPTER OVERVIEW

Thoughts can enter our consciousness uninvited and unplanned, and they wield a great influence over the bodymind. Both positive and negative thoughts and images can affect all body systems as well as physical and mental activity levels and expectations. Overcoming nonproductive lifelong behaviors can be challenging, but with careful choices of interventions and support from others, one can achieve health-affirming change.

## PROCESS EXERCISE NO. 16

(15-minute opening experiential session using music and healing objects if desired.)

### Vision of Healing: Changing Outcomes

Gently helping ourselves identify discrepancies between thoughts and reality allows us to bring the world into a clearer focus. By examining the silent dialogue that accompanies every interaction with the outer world and identifying false assumptions, distortions, and misinterpretations, we can choose to make healthy changes.

Begin with a guided relaxation exercise (5 minutes) and gradually fade in music of choice. Suggest to students that they can close their eyes or leave their eyes open. Ask students who leave their eyes open to focus on a spot several feet in front of them. This allows for a greater ease in following the relaxation and imagery suggestions and reflective experience.

Using techniques for empowering relaxation and imagery scripts (see Chapters 21 and 22), gently weave into a guided imagery exercise reflective questions about the warning signals of stress. Explore the physical responses, automatic thoughts, moods and emotions, exaggerated beliefs, and behaviors associated with the situation. For each situation, describe a more effective response and the potential outcomes of this response. Engage students in feeling the internal experience within during the restructuring. Bring closure to the imagery process.

With soft music still playing, invite students to record in a personal journal (3 to 5 minutes) any images, process questions and answers, or insight gained. Ask students to bring personal closure to this process. Gradually fade music out. Engage students in a gentle stretching exercise before the theory session begins.

## KEY CONCEPTS: THEORY AND RESEARCH

(1-hour presentation)
**OPTIONAL: GUEST SPEAKER(S) AND VIDEO(S)**

**Guest Speaker(s):** Invite one or more nurses experienced in cognitive therapies. Provide guest speaker(s) with the Instructor's Manual suggestions so the speaker(s) can become familiar with the students' assignment before class.

**Video(s):** Show a video of a practitioner who describes, demonstrates, and integrates cognitive therapies (rent from local video store or media catalogue or purchase for school video library). Following the video presentation, ask students for their reactions and comments. Discuss the video and answer questions.

**Definitions:** Review definitions and incorporate into presentation.

**Cognitive Therapy:** Review the theory, history, and research related to cognitive therapy. Describe the basic principles, goals, and process of cognitive therapy.

**Effects of Cognition on Health and Illness:** Describe the bio-psycho-social-spiritual effects of stress.

**Application of the General Principles of Cognitive Therapy:** Describe the applications of cognitive therapy in inpatient and out-patient settings.

## HOLISTIC CARING PROCESS

Focus on specifics of assessment, patterns/challenges/needs, outcomes, therapeutic care plan, implementation, and evaluation. Instruct students in the importance of developing their own style of preparation before, at the beginning of, during, and at the end of the session.

## EXPERIENTIAL EXERCISES

(2 hours. Incorporation of sharing circles and experiential exercises is encouraged in class presentation.)

**Identification of Cognitive Distortions:** Have students work in dyads to uncover a cognitive distortion and identify the thoughts and feelings related to the stress trigger. Next, have them restructure or reframe the distortion to choose a more effective way of coping. Have students share these distortions and restructurings with the group.

**Developing Affirmations:** Have students work in dyads to identify personal behaviors that they wish to change. Have students decide what they want to have happen or how they wish to feel in the situation. Ask students to formulate this goal as an affirmation (first-person statement). Have each student repeat his or her affirmation often during the day and share the experience with others.

**Case Study:** Have students discuss case studies as well as incorporate a case study into group presentation. Encourage students to share other client/patient stories and to focus on the meaning of the stories, symptoms, illness, and use of specific symbols and metaphors.

## DIRECTIONS FOR FUTURE RESEARCH

Have students choose one or more research questions as an area to explore; students should review the literature, identify research findings that could be utilized in practice, and/or postulate additional research questions or hypotheses. Consult with a nurse researcher to help develop a research study. Encourage students to begin collecting articles that can support further investigation.

## NURSE HEALER REFLECTIONS

Encourage students to use the chapter reflective questions as a guide to journal entries for exploring, understanding, and validating presence and healing.

Chapter 17

# Self-Reflection: Consulting the Truth Within

## CHAPTER OBJECTIVES

Refer to chapter for specific theoretical, clinical, and personal objectives. These will provide guidelines for the integration of objectives in class presentation, experiential sessions, and student homework assignments.

## CHAPTER OVERVIEW

Self-reflection interventions are strategies for discovering one's inner wisdom, which is often buried during daily routines. These interventions differ from most client education modules in that the learning comes from inner knowledge and is primarily client-generated. These strategies assist all individuals to reach for higher levels of wellness and understanding of the life process. Self-reflection can be successfully woven into the fabric of both professional and personal life.

## PROCESS EXERCISE NO. 17

(15-minute opening experiential session using music and healing objects if desired.)

### Vision of Healing: Healthy Disclosure

As nurses, we can refresh our own self-reflection techniques and perfect new ones to help us record and grow from our experiences, intuitions, and connections. Self-reflection helps us to evoke more trust and truth in daily life.

Begin with a guided relaxation exercise (5 minutes) and gradually fade in music of choice. Suggest to students that they can close their eyes or leave their eyes open. Ask students who leave their eyes open to focus on a spot several feet in front of them. This allows for a greater ease in following the relaxation and imagery suggestions and reflective experience.

Using techniques for empowering relaxation and imagery scripts (see Chapters 21 and 22), gently weave into a guided imagery exercise the parable in the Vision of Healing. Using the metaphors from the parable, create several reflective questions about truth and invite each student to access and explore a deep truth that is important in his or her life. Bring closure to the imagery process.

With soft music still playing, invite students to record in a personal journal (3 to 5 minutes) any images, process questions and answers, or insight gained. Ask students to bring personal closure to this process. Gradually fade music out. Engage students in a gentle stretching exercise before the theory session begins.

## KEY CONCEPTS: THEORY AND RESEARCH

(1-hour presentation)
OPTIONAL: GUEST SPEAKER(S) AND VIDEO(S)

**Guest Speaker(s):** Invite one or more nurses experienced in self-reflection interventions. Provide guest speaker(s) with the Instructor's Manual suggestions so speaker(s) can become familiar with the students' assignment before class.

**Video(s):** Show a video of a practitioner who describes, demonstrates, and integrates one or more of the self-reflection therapies (rent from a media catalogue or purchase for school video library). Following the video presentation, ask students for their reactions and comments. Discuss the video and answer questions.

**Definitions:** Review definitions and incorporate into presentation.

**Self:** Provide a broad overview of self-reflection. Review the four ways in which adults learn and discuss how the adult learning process differs from the learning process for children. Incorporate within the discussion self-concept, experience, problem solving, and applicability of knowledge.

**Self-Identity:** Discuss self-identity according to Erikson's theory.

**Self-Awareness:** Explore the concept that, to optimize one's personal development as well as one's health and well-being, one must be fully aware of the self.

**Body-Mind-Spirit Connections:** Review how self-reflection acts as an intermediary between the various aspects and expressions of the bodymind. Discuss specific hemispheric function and the importance of both logical and nonlogical ways of knowing.

## HOLISTIC CARING PROCESS

Focus on specifics of assessment, patterns/challenges/needs, outcomes, therapeutic care plan, intervention, and evaluation (Exhibits 17–1 and 17–2). Instruct students in the importance of developing their own style of preparation before, at the beginning of, during, and at the end of the session.

## EXPERIENTIAL EXERCISES

(2 hours. Incorporation of sharing circles and experiential exercises is encouraged in class presentation. Refer to the chapter section entitled "Specific Interventions" for details.)

**Keeping Diaries and Journals:** Prior to this class, have students select a special writing pen, paper, or notebook that will be brought to and used in each class session as well as used for the journaling assignment (5 minutes each day) out of class. Encourage students to explore Progoff's categories and divisions for keeping a journal. Explore the usefulness of a structured client diary and discuss how individuals can gain insight into symptom patterns, healing (or negative) thoughts and images, the impact of interventions used, and the amount of pain medications taken in relationship to daily events.

**Creating Works of Art:** Name different art forms and discuss why the nurse helps the client identify the purpose of the activity in terms of process rather than product.

**Writing Letters:** Have students write a letter to another person that expresses some deep emotions that may have been kept inside (e.g., unconditional love, forgiveness, remembrances, anger, disappointment, etc.).

**Beginning an Intuition Log:** Encourage each student to carry a small notebook in his or her pocket and to record each time the student has a hunch or flash of insight, hears a quiet, inner voice, or senses a vague impression or feeling. Have students share some insights in the next class session.

**Using Metaphors:** Explain how using a metaphor can help a client examine the meaning of a problem. Have students give some examples.

**Learning from Dreams:** Review the reflective questions about dream content for interpretation and clarification. Invite students to practice the lucid dreaming guidelines during the semester. Encourage students to keep a portion of a personal journal for dreams.

**Building Mind Maps and Clusters:** Review the process of clustering (Figure 17–2). Have students work in small groups. In the center of a piece of paper, write the words *healing environment*. Next, have students create a mind map and clusters for a healing environment on another piece of paper. Ask the students to identify areas of their lives, projects, or relationships in which they feel stuck. Ask them to create a cluster of ways to increase creativity and problem solving (e.g., people, ideas, solutions, etc.).

**Using the Mandala and Focusing:** Have students work in dyads to design and describe a mandala that would work for them. Ask them to spend a few minutes focusing on their creation.

**Sharing Stories:** Have students work in triads and, beginning with "Once upon a time," tell a story about an actual event or one created in the moment. Provide time for sharing stories.

**Reminiscing and Embarking on a Life Review:** Explore the life review process. Prior to this class, ask students to do a life review with a child and with a senior citizen. Search for similarities and differences between the reviews of children and those of older adults.

**Case Study:** Have students discuss case studies as well as incorporate a case study into group presentation. Encourage students to share other client/patient stories and to focus on the meaning of symptoms, disease, illness, and use of specific symbols and metaphors.

## DIRECTIONS FOR FUTURE RESEARCH

Have students choose one or more research questions as an area to explore; students should review the literature, identify research findings that could be utilized in practice, and/or postulate additional research questions or hypotheses. Consult with a nurse researcher to help develop a research study.

## NURSE HEALER REFLECTIONS

Encourage students to use the chapter reflective questions as a guide to journal entries for exploring, understanding, and validating presence and healing.

# Chapter 18

# Nutrition

## CHAPTER OBJECTIVES

Refer to chapter for specific theoretical, clinical, and personal objectives. These will provide guidelines for the integration of objectives in class presentation, experiential sessions, and student homework assignments.

## CHAPTER OVERVIEW

Joy and vitality can come from knowing what to eat and what not to eat, preparing healthy foods, having good digestion, and sharing the communal experience of the meal. Poor eating habits due to the lack of knowledge about healthy eating can be a major risk factor for disease. As nurses better understand the challenges and dynamics of nutrition, they can more effectively assess clients, assist them with lifestyle changes, and provide them with guidelines to sustain healthier lifestyle habits.

## PROCESS EXERCISE NO. 18

(15-minute opening experiential session using music and healing objects if desired.)

### Vision of Healing: Nourishing the Bodymind

Nutrition is one of the major keys to promoting high-level wellness. Food consumption, digestion, and elimination have a direct effect on the body-mind-spirit. In general, the feeling of well-being that comes from physical health permeates all of our activities, enables quicker thinking, allows for more restful sleep, and facilitates relaxation that leads to a deeper spiritual understanding.

Begin with a guided relaxation exercise (5 minutes) and gradually fade in music of choice. Suggest to students that they can close their eyes or leave their eyes open. Ask students who leave their eyes open to focus on a spot several feet in front of them. This allows for a greater ease in following the relaxation and imagery suggestions and reflective experience.

Using techniques for empowering relaxation and imagery scripts (see Chapters 21 and 22), gently weave into a guided imagery exercise reflective questions about images of an ideal body that is personally right for the individual. Invite students to imagine standing in front of a mirror and seeing and thinking how they might appear if they were eating at optimal levels. Direct them to consider their body dimensions, strength potential, skin and hair texture, and other aspects that relate directly to nutrition. Bring closure to the imagery process.

With soft music still playing, invite students to record in a personal journal (3 to 5 minutes) any images, process questions and answers, or insight gained. Ask students to bring personal closure to this process. Gradually fade music out. Engage students in a gentle stretching exercise before the theory session begins.

## KEY CONCEPTS: THEORY AND RESEARCH

(1-hour presentation)

**OPTIONAL: GUEST SPEAKER(S) AND VIDEO(S)**

**Guest Speaker(s):** Invite one or more nurses experienced in nutrition counseling. Provide the guest speaker(s) with the Instructor's Manual suggestions so the speaker(s) can become familiar with the students' assignment before class.

**Video(s):** Show a video of a practitioner who describes, demonstrates, and integrates optimal nutrition (rent from media catalogue or purchase for school video library). Following the video presentation, ask students for their reactions and comments. Discuss the video and answer questions.

**Definitions:** Review definitions and incorporate into presentation.

**Theory and Research about Nutrition:** Review current concepts and research findings in the areas of general nutrition, chronic disease and food, food and diseases such as cancer and osteoporosis, and nutrition for populations with special needs, such as older adults and athletes.

**Current Nutritional Recommendations:** Discuss the food guide pyramid and the Mediterranean diet pyramid (Figure 18–1). Compare and contrast these two good guides. Discuss the dietary goals and recommendations described in the chapter.

**Vitamins and Minerals:** Review the recommendations for intake of vitamins and minerals as shown in Tables 18–2 and 18–3.

**Eating to Promote Health:** Review healthy eating guidelines to promote health and reduce risk of cardiovascular diseases, cancer, and osteoporosis.

**Obesity:** Discuss why obesity is one of the most common contemporary health risk factors and examine general guidelines nurses can use in directing clients to reverse their weight gains.

**Healthy Choices in Nutrition:** Review which foods to choose and which ones to avoid.

## HOLISTIC CARING PROCESS

Focus on specifics of assessment, patterns/challenges/needs, outcomes, therapeutic care plan, implementation, and evaluation (Exhibits 18-1 and 18-2). Instruct students in the importance of developing their own style of preparation before, at the beginning of, during, and at the end of the session.

## EXPERIENTIAL EXERCISES

(2 hours. Incorporation of sharing circles and experiential exercises is encouraged for class presentation. Refer to chapter section entitled "Specific Interventions" for details.)

**Assessment of Where I Am Now:** Often we cannot remember what or how much we ate even as recently as yesterday. Before we can adequately assess how well we are addressing our nutritional needs, we need to examine our past behaviors. Ask students to refer to homework assignments on self-assessments and the Circle of Human Potential (Chapter 15).

**Cholesterol-Lowering Diet:** Ask students to review the cholesterol-lowering diet. Discuss how the cholesterol-lowering diet can be incorporated into a personal dietary plan. Explore different teaching strategies for promoting decreased fat intake.

**Case Study:** Have students discuss case studies as well as incorporate a case study into group presentation. Encourage students to share other client/patient stories and to focus on the meaning of the symptoms, disease, illness, and use of specific symbols and metaphors.

## DIRECTIONS FOR FUTURE RESEARCH

Have students choose one or more research questions as an area to explore; students should review the literature, identify research findings that could be utilized in practice, and/or postulate additional research questions or hypotheses. Consult with a nurse researcher to help develop a research study. Encourage students to begin collecting articles that can support further investigation.

## NURSE HEALER REFLECTIONS

Encourage students to use the chapter reflective questions as a guide to journal entries for exploring, understanding, and validating presence and healing.

# Chapter 19

# Exercise and Movement

## CHAPTER OBJECTIVES

Refer to chapter for specific theoretical, clinical, and personal objectives. These will assist with the integration of objectives in class presentation, experiential sessions, and student homework assignments

## CHAPTER OVERVIEW

Strength, flexibility, and a sense of well-being can come from exercising regularly and moving creatively to the rhythm of life. The lack of these health habits can be major risk factors for disease. As nurses better understand the challenges and dynamics of exercise and movement, they can more effectively assess clients, assist them with lifestyle changes, and provide them with guidelines to sustain healthier lifestyle habits.

## PROCESS EXERCISE NO. 19

(15-minute opening experiential session using music and healing objects if desired.)

### Vision of Healing: Strengthening the Bodymind

Exercise and movement work synergistically to promote high-level wellness. The amount and quality of physical activity has a direct effect on the body-mind-spirit. The feeling of well-being that comes from physical health permeates all of our activities, enabling quicker thinking, allowing for more restful sleep, and facilitating relaxation that leads to a deeper spiritual understanding.

Begin with a guided relaxation exercise (5 minutes) and gradually fade in music of choice. Suggest to students that they can close their eyes or leave them open. Ask students who leave their eyes open to focus on a spot several feet in front of them. This allows for a greater ease in following the relaxation and imagery suggestions and reflective experience.

Using techniques for empowering relaxation and imagery scripts (see Chapters 21 and 22), gently weave into a guided imagery exercise reflective questions about images of an ideal body that is personally right for the individual.

Invite students to imagine standing in front of a mirror and seeing and thinking how they might appear if they were exercising and moving at optimal levels. Direct them to consider their body dimensions, posture, flexibility, strength potential, and other aspects that directly relate to movement and exercise. Bring closure to the imagery process.

With soft music still playing, invite students to record in a personal journal (3 to 5 minutes) any images, process questions and answers, or insight gained. Ask students to bring personal closure to this process. Gradually fade music out. Engage students in a gentle stretching exercise before the theory session begins.

## KEY CONCEPTS: THEORY AND RESEARCH

(1-hour presentation)

**OPTIONAL: GUEST SPEAKER(S) AND VIDEOS**

**Guest Speaker(s):** Invite one or more nurses experienced in exercise and movement counseling. Provide the great speaker(s) with the Instructor's Manual suggestions so the speaker(s) can become familiar with the students' assignments before class.

**Video(s):** Show a video of a practitioner who describes, demonstrates, and integrates exercise and movement (rent from media catalogue or purchase for school video library). Following the video presentation, ask students for their reactions and comments. Discuss the video and answer questions.

**Definitions:** Review definitions and incorporate into presentation.

**Exercise:** Discuss traditional exercise programs and the reasons that exercise is important in the maintenance of health.

**Exercise Needs in Special Situations:** Review exercise needs in special situations, for special population groups, and for certain health conditions—AIDS, cardiovascular disease, diabetes, neuromuscular conditions, orthopedic conditions, osteoporosis, respiratory disease, rheumatic disease, and psychiatric conditions.

**Movement:** Review movement therapies and discuss how they can broaden the scope and choices of available exercise programs.

## HOLISTIC CARING PROCESS

Focus on specifics of assessment, patterns/challenges/needs, outcomes, therapeutic care plan, implementation, and evaluation (Exhibits 19–1 and 19–2). Instruct students in the importance of developing their own style of preparation before, at the beginning of, during, and at the end of a session.

## EXPERIENTIAL EXERCISES

(2 hours. Incorporation of sharing circles and experiential exercises is encouraged for class presentation. Refer to chapter section entitled "Specific Interventions" for details.)

**Assessment of Where I Am Now:** Often we cannot remember our exact activities or how much movement we incorporated into our lives even as recently as yesterday. Before we can adequately assess how well we are addressing our exercise needs, we need to examine our past behaviors. Ask students to refer to homework assignments on self-assessments and the Circle of Human Potentials (Chapter 15).

**Exercise:** Review the three key points of an exercise program. Ask students to self-design a program that will work for them. Consider how and in what setting information on exercise is introduced to clients.

**Movement:** Review the four components of creative movement: centering, warm-up, exploration of surrounding space, and stretching. Incorporate stretching and movement exercises in class.

**Case Study:** Have students discuss case studies as well as incorporate a case study into group presentation. Encourage students to share other client/patient stories and to focus on the meaning of the symptoms, disease, illness, and use of specific symbols and metaphors.

## DIRECTIONS FOR FUTURE RESEARCH

Have students choose one or more research questions as an area to explore; students should review the literature, identify the research findings that could be utilized in practice, and/or postulate additional research questions or hypotheses. Consult with a nurse researcher to help develop a research study. Encourage students to help develop a research study. Encourage students to begin collecting articles that can support further investigation.

## NURSE HEALER REFLECTIONS

Encourage students to use the chapter reflective questions as a guide to journal entries for exploring, understanding, and validating presence and healing.

Chapter 20

# Humor, Laughter, and Play: Maintaining Balance in a Serious World

## CHAPTER OBJECTIVES

Refer to chapter for specific theoretical, clinical, and person objectives. These will provide guidelines for the integration of objectives in class presentation, experiential sessions, and student homework assignments.

## CHAPTER OVERVIEW

Whether we are guiding ourselves or our clients through difficult procedures or strengthening our ability to move smoothly through a shift assignment, humor and playfulness help keep us centered and whole. Humor can help us tap into the spiritual and evolutionary possibilities inherent in all events.

## PROCESS EXERCISE NO. 20

(15-minute opening experiential session using music and healing objects if desired.)

### Vision of Healing: Releasing the Energy of the Playful Child

Play is part of the richness of life; it enables us to live and grow. As infants and children we play to learn. As adults, we play to relax, to enjoy interaction with others, to grow, and to gain a different perspective on our lives. Our play can encompass a variety of activities, from the simple experience of skipping or dancing for the joy of movement to the excitement of playing to win in a tournament or game.

Begin with a guided relaxation exercise (5 minutes) and gradually fade in music of choice. Suggest to students that they can close their eyes or leave their eyes open. Ask students who leave their eyes open to focus on a spot several feet in front of them. This allows for a greater ease in following the relaxation and imagery suggestions and reflective experience.

Using techniques for empowering relaxation and imagery scripts (see Chapters 21 and 22), gently weave into a guided imagery exercise reflective questions that prompt students to remember an event or time in which spontaneous hilarity was present. Encourage them to engage in the moment, remembering as many details as possible and using all of their senses. Invite them to laugh out loud as they evoke this special memory. Bring closure to the imagery process.

With soft music still playing, invite students to record in a personal journal (3 to 5 minutes) any images, process questions and answers, or insight gained. Ask students to bring personal closure to this process. Gradually fade music out. Engage students in a gentle stretching exercise before the theory session begins.

## KEY CONCEPTS: THEORY AND RESEARCH

(1-hour presentation)

OPTIONAL: GUEST SPEAKER(S) AND VIDEO(S)

**Guest Speaker(s):** Invite a nurse and/or clown experienced in play and laughter therapies. Provide guest speaker(s) with the Instructor's Manual suggestions so the speaker(s) can become familiar with the students' assignment before class.

**Video(s):** Show a video that evokes play and laughter (rent from local video store or media catalogue or purchase for school video library). Following the video presentation, ask students for their reactions and comments. Discuss the video and answer questions.

**Definitions:** Review definitions and incorporate into presentation.

**Humor from Different Perspectives:** Discuss comedy and laughter from the time of the ancient Greeks to the present. Discuss how psychoanalytic theory views joking.

**Therapeutic Humor:** Review the research on play and laughter and their relationship to health and healing.

**Hoping Humor—Courage to Face Challenges:** Discuss how the ability to hope for something better enables human beings to face difficult situations. Give an example.

**Coping Humor—Release for Tension:** Examine how play and laughter allow individuals to forgive themselves for imperfections, mistakes, and failures.

**Sounds of Laughter:** Examine how different kinds of laughter reflect different internal states of being.

**Physiologic Response to Laughter:** Review how laughter affects physiology. Give examples.

**The Power of Playfulness:** Review how the ancients used play. Explore how a shift in attitude at work can allow an individual to feel freedom and to "recharge the battery."

**Humor and Stress Management:** Explore how and why humor exists and how to use it to effectively manage stress.

**Humor and Locus of Control:** Review the research on the relationship between humor and locus of control.

## HOLISTIC CARING PROCESS

Focus on specifics of assessment, patterns/challenges/needs, outcomes, therapeutic care plan, implementation, and evaluation (Exhibits 20–2 and 20–4). Instruct students in the importance of developing their own style of preparation before, at the beginning of, during, and at the end of the session.

## EXPERIENTIAL EXERCISES

(2 hours. Incorporation of sharing circles and experiential exercises is encouraged in class presentation. Refer to chapter section entitled "Specific Interventions" for details.)

**Cultivating Spontaneous Silliness:** Have students work in dyads and identify times during the day when they play with a sense of freedom and without guilt, rather than competing.

**Playing Games:** Have students work in groups of three to five people and spontaneously come up with a game in a few minutes. For example, practice laughing out loud until a deep, clear belly laugh is heard from everyone. Then engage the rest of the class in the playfulness of the game. Share in a group the play strategies used in a day to decrease the stress of responsibility and work.

**Collecting Cartoons:** Prior to this class, ask students to collect a few cartoons that are humorous. Spend time in class sharing cartoons and assess the variety of humor and satire.

**Using Humorous Books, Audiotapes, and Video:** Prior to this class, review at least one humorous book, audiotape, or video. Bring a reference to class and explore the ease with which a group can create a humor library. Discuss the articles to be included, determine the categories into which they can be placed, and decide whether specific items might be more effective for certain groups of clients or patients.

**Case Study:** Have students discuss case studies as well as incorporate a case study into group presentation. Encourage students to share other client/patient stories and to focus on the meaning of the stories, symptoms, and illness, and the use of specific symbols and metaphors.

## DIRECTIONS FOR FUTURE RESEARCH

Have students choose one or more research questions as an area to explore; students should review the literature, identify research findings that could be utilized in practice, and/or postulate additional research questions or hypotheses. Consult with a nurse researcher to help develop a research study. Encourage students to begin collecting articles that can support further investigation.

## NURSE HEALER REFLECTIONS

Encourage students to use the chapter reflective questions as a guide to journal entries for exploring, understanding, and validating presence and healing.

# Chapter 21

# Relaxation: The First Step to Restore, Renew, and Self-Heal

## CHAPTER OBJECTIVES

Refer to chapter for specific theoretical, clinical, and personal objectives. These will assist with the integration of objectives in class presentation, experiential sessions, and student homework assignments.

## CHAPTER OVERVIEW

Relaxation calms the bodymind and helps us to focus inward. Regardless of the approach used, the end result is a movement of the person toward balance and healing. Relaxation exercises can be taught under almost any circumstances. These interventions not only can reduce the fear and anxiety associated with medical and nursing procedures but, once learned, can be used in all aspects of a client's life.

## PROCESS EXERCISE NO. 21

(15-minute opening experiential session using music and healing objects if desired.)

### Vision of Healing: Creating Receptive Quiet

Learning to create a state of mindfulness in which there is an absence of physical, mental, and emotional tension is an important healing technique. As the skill of being in the present moment is cultivated, we have greater opportunities to move toward wholeness and well-being.

Begin with a guided relaxation exercise (5 minutes) and gradually fade in music of choice. Suggest to students that they can close their eyes or leave their eyes open. Ask students who leave their eyes open to focus on a spot several feet in front of them. This allows for a greater ease in following the relaxation and imagery suggestions and reflective experience.

Using techniques for empowering relaxation and imagery scripts (see also Chapters 21 and 22), gently weave reflective questions into a guided imagery exercise as the power of the healing rhythm of relaxed breathing is explored. Bring closure to the imagery process.

With soft music still playing, invite students to record in a personal journal (3 to 5 minutes) any images, process questions and answers, or insight gained. Ask students to bring personal closure to this process. Gradually fade music out. Engage students in a gentle stretching exercise before the theory session begins.

## KEY CONCEPTS: THEORY AND RESEARCH

(1-hour presentation)

**OPTIONAL: GUEST SPEAKER(S) AND VIDEO(S)**

**Guest Speaker(s):** Invite a nurse or professional who uses biofeedback to demonstrate biofeedback procedures. Give students an opportunity to use the biofeedback equipment and to incorporate relaxation and imagery techniques while using the equipment. Provide the guest speaker with the Instructor's Manual suggestions so the speaker can become familiar with the students' assignment before class.

**Video(s):** Show a video that demonstrates use of relaxation, self-hypnosis, or biofeedback (rent from a media catalogue or purchase for school library). Following the video presentation, ask students for their reactions and comments. Discuss the video and answer questions.

**Definitions:** Review definitions and incorporate into presentation.

**Relaxation:** Discuss the general definition, ancient uses, and indications for relaxation. Explore the clinical application of various relaxation techniques in practice.

**The Stress Response:** Explore the various psychophysiologic responses to stress.

**The Relaxation Response:** Explore the body-mind-spirit effects of relaxation.

**Breathing and Energy Healing Practice:** Discuss various breathing and energy healing practices.

**Meditation:** Compare and contrast various meditation practices.

**Modern Methods Relation:** Compare and contrast various modern forms of relaxation outlined in Table 21–2.

**Selecting Relaxation Interventions for Clients:** Review strategies for individualizing relaxation interventions for clients.

**Hypnosis and Self-Hypnosis:** Explore how hypnosis and self-hypnosis can be used for healing and therapeutic purposes.

**Biofeedback:** Explore the use of biofeedback for relaxation and healing.

**Cautions and Contraindications for Relaxation, Meditation, and Biofeedback:** Discuss various cautions and contraindications for relaxation interventions.

PTSD: Discuss elements of post-traumatic stress disorder and perspectives for living in a time of uncertainty.

**Restorative Practices:** Compare and contrast various restorative practices.

## HOLISTIC CARING PROCESS

Focus on specifics of assessment, patterns/challenges/needs, outcomes, therapeutic care plan, implementation, and evaluation (Exhibits 21–8 and 21–9). Instruct students in the importance of developing their own style of preparation before, at the beginning of, during, and at the end of the session.

## EXPERIENTIAL EXERCISES

(2 hours. Incorporation of sharing circles and experiential exercises is encouraged in class presentation.)

**Relaxation Interventions:** Prior to this class, ask students to pick one or a combination of breathing techniques and apply them during stressful moments for 1 week. Have students share new skills for promoting increased awareness of where tension accumulates in the body during stressful moments.

Have students work in dyads and guide each other in general breathing exercises, progressive muscle relaxation, and autogenic training. Discuss the experience of being the guide and the experience of being the recipient of relaxation strategies; examine what worked best and what worked least while being guided in each intervention.

**Meditation:** Ask students to sit and meditate for a 20-minute period. Share how quieting the mind is a challenge and requires discipline.

**Prayer:** Encourage students to write or read a short prayer and to focus on the inward experience of moving into a contemplative state of being. Explore the faith factor that occurs with relaxation, particularly when individuals choose their own prayer.

**Biofeedback:** If a guest speaker is not part of the class, visit a biofeedback laboratory. Provide students with an opportunity to use the biofeedback equipment to experience constant feedback with various degrees of relaxation. Have each student identify a piece of equipment commonly used in nursing practice and describe how it could be used as a biofeedback device.

**Hypnosis and Self-Hypnosis:** Investigate the differences in hypnosis and self-hypnosis. Ask students to recognize negative self-talk and to create a healthier self-talk dialogue. Have students recount a clinical situation in which they assisted a client in identifying negative self-talk and then helped the client construct a healthier self-talk.

**Case Study:** Have students discuss case studies involving relaxation interventions as well as incorporate a case study into group presentation. Encourage students to share other client/patient stories and to focus on the meaning of symptoms, disease, illness, and use of specific symbols and metaphors.

## DIRECTIONS FOR FUTURE RESEARCH

Have students choose one or more research questions as an area to explore; students should review the literature, identify research findings that could be utilized in practice, and/or postulate additional research questions or hypotheses. Consult with a nurse researcher to help develop a research study. Encourage students to begin collecting articles that can support further investigation.

## NURSE HEALER REFLECTIONS

Encourage students to use the chapter reflective questions as a guide to journal entries for exploring, understanding, and validating presence and healing.

Chapter 22

# Imagery: Awakening the Inner Healer

## CHAPTER OBJECTIVES

Refer to chapter for specific theoretical, clinical, and personal objectives. These will provide guidelines for the integration of objectives in class presentation, experiential sessions, and student homework assignments.

## CHAPTER OVERVIEW

Imagery is the most ancient and potent healing resource in the history of medicine. Through our senses, imagery creates the interface between body, mind, and spirit. It is like a midwife, assisting the birth of conscious expression from the depths of inner experience. Imagery is an essential aspect of holistic nursing practice.

## PROCESS EXERCISE NO. 22

(15-minute opening experiential session using music and other healing objects if desired.)

### Vision of Healing: Modeling a Wellness Lifestyle

Self-assessment is an essential step in modeling a wellness lifestyle. Ask students to reflect on their self-assessments and the Circle of Human Potential (Chapter 15).

Begin with a guided relaxation exercise (5 minutes) and gradually fade in music of choice. Suggest to students that they can close their eyes or leave their eyes open. Ask students who leave their eyes open to focus on a spot several feet in front of them. This allows for a greater ease in following the relaxation and imagery suggestions and reflective experience.

Using techniques for empowering relaxation and imagery scripts (see also Chapter 21), gently weave into a guided imagery exercise reflective questions about where students are in their lives at this time. Have them reflect on the areas of self-assessment, any desired change, the requirements for change, and attitudes, beliefs, and support systems. Ask students to go forward in time to the next hour and to experience in their imagination modeling and living the Circle of Human Potential as imagery suggestions about each area are slowly integrated. Bring closure to the imagery process.

With soft music still playing, invite students to record in a personal journal (3 to 5 minutes) any images, process questions and answers, or insight gained. Ask students to bring personal closure to this process. Gradually fade music out. Engage students in a gentle stretching exercise before the theory session begins.

## KEY CONCEPTS: THEORY AND RESEARCH

(1-hour presentation)

**OPTIONAL: GUEST SPEAKER(S) AND VIDEO(S)**

**Guest Speaker(s):** Invite one or more nurses experienced in the use of imagery in clinical practice or an art therapist. Provide guest speaker(s) with the Instructor's Manual suggestions so the speaker(s) can become familiar with the students' assignment before class.

**Video(s):** Show a video of a practitioner describing and demonstrating one or more imagery modalities in clinical practice (rent from media catalogue or purchase for school video library). Following the video presentation, ask students for their reactions and comments. Discuss the video and answer questions.

**Definitions:** Review definitions and incorporate into presentation.

**Introduction to Imagery:** Increase the students' awareness of the senses. Have students become aware of how each sense, when stimulated, can enhance another sense. Incorporating an experiential imagery exercise with the theoretical presentation is very effective.

**Imagery and States of Consciousness:** Explore research findings regarding the ongoing imagery process, or streams of consciousness.

**Clinical Effectiveness of Imagery:** Discuss specific clinical studies showing the effectiveness of imagery in managing certain symptoms, illnesses, and diseases.

**Clinical Imagery Theories:** Review the two theories discussed. Use the example of a worry or a fear (test anxiety, concerns regarding money, relationships, time, complications of surgery, etc.) as each theory is analyzed to demonstrate how an individual can create a new healing image in self-dialogue and imagery rehearsal. Connect theories with different types of imagery in experiential session.

**Clinical Techniques in Imagery:** Discuss clinical techniques used in imagery. Reinforce that one or more of the senses is used in all of these imagery patterns.

**Imagery in Holistic Health Counseling:** Explore the use of imagery in healing relationships.

**Values and Spirituality:** Discuss the effective use of imagery in exploring one's values and spirituality, and in making lifestyle choices.

**Transpersonal Imagery:** Explore the concept of transpersonal imagery and its effectiveness in holistic nursing practice. Explore the use of symbols and metaphors of transformation (Table 22–1).

**Imagery with Disease/Illness:** Discuss the concrete experiences (subjective and objective experiences) that clients/patients undergo during tests and procedures. Review documented descriptors of subjective experience during stressful events (Table 22–2). Have students add to this list. Describe sensations evoked by selected procedures as documented in the literature.

**Fears in Imagery Work:** Discuss three predictable and understandable fears encountered in imagery work: that nothing will happen; that too much will happen; and that it will be done incorrectly.

## HOLISTIC CARING PROCESS

Focus on specifics of assessment, patterns/challenges/needs, outcomes, therapeutic care plan, implementation, and evaluation for imagery (Exhibit 22-1 and Table 22-3). Instruct students in the importance of developing their own style of preparation before, at the beginning of, during, and at the end of the session.

## EXPERIENTIAL EXERCISES

(2 hours. Incorporation of sharing circles and experiential exercises is encouraged in class presentation.)

**Facilitation and Interpretation of the Imagery Process:** Encourage students in daily journaling to record their own images of stress symptoms and the personal meaning of these symptoms.

Share different client/patient images and describe how the client/patient interpreted the symptoms, worries, or fears. To elicit these images, encourage students to use the technique for empowering the spoken word. Refer to the guidelines for teaching the imagery process of identifying the problem/disease, the inner healing resources, and the external healing resources.

Coach students in how to guide others in a general imagery exercise. Throughout the course have students briefly share their experiences and personal dominant sensory modalities with different exercises. Ask students to experience the following with eyes closed:

*Touch:* Place hands on lap and feel texture of clothing on skin. What images or memories come?

*Hearing:* Sound a chime or bell. What images and memories come?

*Vision:* Focus on a special color in the mind's eye. What images or memories come?

*Smell:* Imagine the smell of vanilla. What images or memories come?

*Taste:* Imagine a lemon. Feel its texture. Now cut and smell the lemon. Imagine a drop of lemon juice on the tongue. Notice increased salivation. Just thinking about this experience produces what kind of imagery sensations? What images or memories come?

*Kinesthesia:* What inner experiences occur with stimulation of the kinesthetic sense? What images or memories come?

Guide students in or coach students in how to guide a relaxation and imagery exercise to identify the different types of imagery. Music will enhance the awareness of the different senses as well as the imagery process.

*Spontaneous Imagery:* Identify where tension is carried in the body. What are your first bodily sensations or inner awareness of the presence of tension? Discover your dominant sensory modality. Take the image of tension and begin to create or change it to a helpful, healing image or sensation.

*Correct Biologic Imagery:* If any current health problem exists, identify images from textbooks, magazines, or drug advertisements that incorporate physiology to better understand the physiology of the problem. Review bone, wound, and burn graft healing images.

*Symbolic Imagery:* Remember that symbolic images emerge from the psyche to evoke healing. These images are one's own hero's journey and personal mythology. These images are influenced by media, art, cartoons, symbols, and fantasy characters. For instance, symbolic images may reflect not only deep-seated past trauma but current discomfort that may also be associated with physical injury or dysfunction. As an example, for neck pain, symbolic images may be knots, knives, pitchforks, and so forth. The healing images would involve release, removal, untying, melting, or whatever seems to work given the nature of the symbolic image. The shift from correct biologic image to symbolic image usually is a dramatic event and often involves one or more of the senses.

*Imagery Rehearsal:* Have students identify a current situation that needs healing and rehearse step-by-step images directed toward the desired outcomes.

*End-State Imagery:* Take the image just identified and imagine it in a final, healed state or rehearse the final outcome desired.

*General Healing Imagery:* Identify a healing image, color, sound, and so on, that has qualities that evoke healing and inner peace.

**Guided Imagery Scripts:** Have students work in dyads in class or out of class using a simple induction technique for imagery. Then have them experience one or more of the specific scripts. Encourage students to share with each other what part of the guiding worked best and what could have been more effective. Follow the guidelines for imagery scripts to enhance the use of imagery as a nursing intervention. Have students use the same interventions with family members or friends to gain more experience.

**Drawing:** Reinforce that the drawing exercise is performed to gain access to internal information of which the individual is not normally aware. Drawing helps the individual to connect with inner healing resources, creativity, and problem-solving. It has nothing to do with one's drawing ability. Using crayons, colored markers, oil pastels, and paper, follow the suggestions given in the textbook for group drawing.

**Disease/Symptom Drawing:** Have each student work with a family member, friend, or client/patient who has symptoms or disease. Follow the guidelines given on helping the individual identify the disease or disability, the internal healing resources, and the external healing resources. Explore the vividness and strength of the internal and external healing resources to eliminate, reverse, or stabilize the symptoms or disease and move the individual toward desired outcomes.

Refer to bone, wound, burn graft, and immune illustrations for examples (Figures 22-1 to 22-4). Reinforce that all client/patient teaching and learning sessions should engage the imagination. As nurses teach clients/patients imagery skills to help them identify their dominant sensory modality, their desired outcomes, the normal physiologic healing process, external healing resources, and internal healing resources, the teaching/learning sessions become much more effective.

**Group Drawing:** Have students identify all the things for which they are thankful or which excite them about life. As each student is given the opportunity to share a personal story, reinforce the healing moment and presence of being listened to by another and emphasize the way that healing occurs in the listening and the telling of a story.

**Case Study:** Have students discuss case studies involving imagery as well as incorporate a case study into group presentation. Encourage students to share other client/patient stories and to focus on the meaning of the symptoms, disease, illness, and use of specific symbols and metaphors.

## DIRECTIONS FOR FUTURE RESEARCH

Have students choose one or more research questions as an area to explore; students should review the literature, identify research findings that could be utilized in practice, and/or postulate additional research questions or hypotheses. Consult with a nurse researcher to help develop a research study. Encourage students to begin collecting articles that can support further investigation.

## NURSE HEALER REFLECTIONS

Encourage students to use the chapter reflective questions as a guide to journal entries for exploring, understanding, and validating presence and healing.

Chapter 23

# Music Therapy: Hearing the Melody of the Soul

## CHAPTER OBJECTIVES

Refer to chapter for specific theoretical, clinical, and personal objectives. These will provide guidelines for the integration of objectives in class presentation, experiential sessions, and student homework assignments.

## CHAPTER OVERVIEW

Music has been a vital part of all societies and cultures, regardless of how primitive or advanced. It is not surprising, then, that music is currently being applied as a complementary therapy in health care. Music therapy is a behavioral science concerned with the use of specific kinds of music to effect changes in behavior, emotions, and physiology. As nurses incorporate music therapy into all areas of clinical practice, they can reduce psychophysiologic stress, anxiety, and pain in clients/patients as well as in their own personal lives.

## PROCESS EXERCISE NO. 23

(15-minute opening experiential session using music and healing objects if desired.)

### Vision of Healing: Composing the Harmony

There is something about the power of music that cannot be expressed in verbal language. Music literally can flow into every cell in the body when one is in a relaxed state.

Begin with a guided relaxation exercise (5 minutes) and gradually fade in music of choice. Suggest to students that they can close their eyes or leave their eyes open. Ask students who leave their eyes open to focus on a spot several feet in front of them. This allows for a greater ease in following the relaxation and imagery suggestions and reflective experience.

Using techniques for empowering relaxation and imagery scripts (see Chapters 21 and 22), gently weave into a guided music exercise reflective questions from the music script Merging the Bodymind with Music. Bring closure to the guided music therapy process.

With soft music still playing, invite students to record in a personal journal (3 to 5 minutes) any images, process questions and answers, or insight gained. Ask students to bring personal closure to this process. Gradually fade music out. Engage students in a gentle stretching exercise before the theory session begins.

## KEY CONCEPTS: THEORY AND RESEARCH

(1-hour presentation)

**OPTIONAL: GUEST SPEAKER(S) AND VIDEO(S)**

**Guest Speaker(s):** Invite a nurse who uses music in clinical practice and/or a music therapist. Provide the guest speaker(s) with the Instructor's Manual suggestions so the speaker(s) can become familiar with the students' assignment before class.

**Video(s):** Show a video that demonstrates the use of music for relaxation or during painful medical or surgical procedures (rent from a media catalogue or purchase for school library). Following the video presentation, ask students for their reactions and comments. Discuss the video and answer questions.

**Definitions:** Review definitions and incorporate into presentation.

**Music Theory and Research:** Review the use of music from a historical perspective.

**Sound, Frequency, and Intensity:** Discuss the principles and theories of sound to understand fully its tremendous capacity to achieve therapeutic psychophysiologic outcomes.

**Purposes of Music Therapy:** Discuss the purposes of music and its application in the clinical setting.

**Psychophysiologic Responses:** Explore the effects of music therapy on shifting states of consciousness, hemispheric functioning, emotions, imagery, the senses, the limbic system, and the human body.

**Music Therapy Applications:** Review the various outcomes that can be achieved with music therapy.

**Music Therapy in Clinical Settings:** Analyze the various patient populations and clinical settings in which music has been used as a healing intervention.

**Selection of Appropriate Music:** Reinforce the importance of selecting the appropriate music for each person; explore various types of music, individual musical preferences, and methods for recording a personal tape.

## HOLISTIC CARING PROCESS

Focus on specifics of assessment, patterns/challenges/needs, outcomes, therapeutic care plan, implementation, and evaluation (Table 23-2 and Exhibit 23-1). Instruct students in the importance of developing their own style of preparation before, at the beginning of, during, and at the end of the session.

## EXPERIENTIAL EXERCISES

(2 hours. Incorporation of sharing circles and experiential exercises is encouraged in class presentation. Refer to chapter section entitled "Specific Interventions" for details.)

**Development of an Audiotape/Videotape Library:** Have students develop an audio/video library for use throughout the semester. Follow the guidelines given for a check-in and check-out procedure.

**Music Therapy Scripts:** Incorporate the music scripts provided in the chapter. Allow time for students to share their experiences with each other. At the end of the session, provide students with paper, crayons, and colored markers for a drawing exercise.

**Case Study:** Have students discuss case studies involving the use of music therapy as well as incorporate a case study into group presentation. Encourage students to share other client/patient stories and to focus on the meaning of symptoms, disease, illness, and use of specific symbols and metaphors.

## DIRECTIONS FOR FUTURE RESEARCH

Have students choose one or more research questions as an area to explore; students should review the literature, identify research findings that could be utilized in practice, and/or postulate additional research questions or hypotheses. Consult with a nurse researcher to help develop a research study. Encourage students to begin collecting articles that can support further investigation.

## NURSE HEALER REFLECTIONS

Encourage students to use the chapter reflective questions as a guide to journal entries for exploring, understanding, and validating presence and healing.

## Chapter 24

# Touch: connecting with the Healing Power

## CHAPTER OBJECTIVES

Refer to chapter for specific theoretical, clinical, and personal objectives. These will provide guidelines for the integration of objectives in class presentation, experiential sessions, and student homework assignments.

## CHAPTER OVERVIEW

Many practitioners and recipients of touch modalities report that the end result shows more benefits than just the obvious advantageous physical effects. Numerous touch therapies have been developed, and are taught and administered by increasing numbers of practitioners. Both direct and indirect body-mind-spirit effects of touch therapies have been demonstrated to enhance healing through one of the body's main sense organs, the skin.

## PROCESS EXERCISE NO. 24

(15-minute opening experiential session using music and healing objects if desired.)

### Vision of Healing: Using Our Healing Hands

Each touch therapy has specific touch skills. Some of these skills are stroking, kneading, manipulation, light touch, pressure point touch, and work within an energy field.

Begin with a guided relaxation exercise (5 minutes) and gradually fade in music of choice. Suggest to students that they can close their eyes or leave their eyes open. Ask students who leave their eyes open to focus on a spot several feet in front of them. This allows for a greater ease in following the relaxation and imagery suggestions and reflective experience.

Using techniques for empowering relaxation and imagery scripts (see Chapters 21 and 22), gently weave into a guided imagery exercise the following reflective questions. What does touch mean to you? How do you feel when you touch an elderly person, a terminally ill child, or someone who seeks stress reduction? Add three to five more reflective questions in regard to touch. Bring closure to the imagery process.

With soft music still playing, invite students to record in a personal journal (3 to 5 minutes) any images, process questions and answers, or insight gained. Ask students to bring personal closure to this process. Gradually fade music out. Engage students in a gentle stretching exercise before the theory session begins.

## KEY CONCEPTS: THEORY AND RESEARCH

(1-hour presentation)
**OPTIONAL: GUEST SPEAKER(S) AND VIDEO(S)**

**Guest Speaker(s):** Invite one or more nurses experienced in touch therapies. Provide guest speaker(s) with the Instructor's Manual suggestions so the speaker(s) can become familiar with the students' reading assignment before class.

**Video(s):** Show a video of a practitioner who describes, demonstrates, and integrates one or more touch modalities (rent from media catalogue or purchase for school video library). Following the video presentation, ask students for their reactions and comments. Discuss the video and answer questions.

**Definitions:** Review definitions and incorporate into presentation.

**Touch in Ancient Times:** Review the multi-thousand-year history of touch. Discuss how massage was used with dream work to prepare individuals for healing during the height of Greek civilization.

**Cultural Variations:** Attitudes toward touch vary from culture to culture and from individual to individual. Encourage students to be sensitive to individual differences and diverse cultural attitudes, such as the view of touch as taboo in one culture and as health enhancing in another culture.

**Validation Studies:** Review clinical research to support the effectiveness of touch therapies in a variety of health care delivery settings.

**Touch Techniques:** Explore how touch is a method of bodymind communication. Discuss the basic techniques of therapeutic massage, Therapeutic Touch, healing touch, acupressure, Shiatzu, and reflexology.

## HOLISTIC CARING PROCESS

Focus on specifics of assessment, patterns/challenges/needs, outcomes, therapeutic care plan, implementation, and evaluation (Exhibits 24–1 and 24–2). Instruct students in the importance of developing their own style of preparation before, at the beginning of, during, and at the end of the session.

## EXPERIENTIAL EXERCISES

(2 hours. Incorporation of sharing circles and experiential exercises is encouraged for class presentation. Refer to the chapter section entitled "Specific Interventions" for details.)

**Touch:** Have students work in dyads and begin the touch experiences. Throughout the exercise have students briefly share their bodymind sensations with their practice partner. Guide the students through the basic therapeutic massage strokes as they apply them to their partner's back. Begin the experience by leading both the giver and the receiver of touch through a series of relaxation steps. For an advanced session, add music and imagery to the exercise.

**Basic Swedish Massage Strokes:** This massage modality is the one used historically in nursing practice. It is most useful for complete bodymind relaxation to evoke sleep or reduce stress, or as stimulating therapy to increase circulation in the bedridden patient.

***Effleurage* (ef-flur-ahj):** A French word meaning to touch lightly. Use this stroke to begin and end the session. This light touch acquaints the recipient with the touch of the practitioner and warms up the area for later strokes. Student practitioner, run your hands along the length of the torso from the neck to the base of the recipient's spine or from the base of the spine up to the base of the neck. Practice using the stroke with the joined tips of the fingers, the palms of the hands, and the ball of the thumb. The increased circulation and increased sweat gland activity moves waste products from inner cellular storage into the bloodstream and out of the body. Feel the rejuvenation of the dermal and epidermal layers of the skin.

***Pétrissage* (pet-ris-ahj):** Student practitioner, with one or both hands, carefully lift up the recipient's muscles along each vertical side of the back, then roll, wring, and squeeze them. Ask the recipient to feel the increasing circulation and to imagine lactic acid moving out of the cells and nutrients passing into the cells, contributing to increasing muscle size and strength.

***Friction*:** Student practitioner, using thumb or fingertips, apply deep, circular movement near the joints and other body areas such as the sides of the spine. Recipient, feel the release of knots that occur when muscle fibers bind together. Become aware that this decrease in muscle tension allows for more flexible joints, tendons, and muscles.

***Tapotement* (tap-ot-maw):** Student practitioner, use this short, chopping movement to chop or hack with the edge of your hand on the recipient. Tap with your fingertips and clap with the palms or the flat surface of your hands and fingers. For a few seconds apply extra stimulation if the recipient has muscle strains or spasms.

***Vibration or shaking:*** Student practitioner, spread your hands or fingers on the recipient's back, press down firmly, and rapidly shake for a few seconds with a trembling motion. Recipient, feel this stroke stimulating the nervous system and increasing the power of the muscles to contract. Focus on how these techniques boost circulation and increase the activities of the glands.

At the end of the session, ask students to exchange impressions about the perceived length of the session, the effectiveness of the exercise, the physical effort on the part of the practitioner, and the degree of relaxation on the part of the recipient. If time permits, ask the partners to switch roles and repeat the steps in this exercise.

**Case Study:** Have students discuss case studies involving the use of touch as well as incorporate a case study into group presentation. Encourage students to share other client/patient stories and to focus on the meaning of the symptoms, disease, illness, and use of specific symbols and metaphors.

## DIRECTIONS FOR FUTURE RESEARCH

Have students choose one or more research questions as an area to explore; students should review the literature, identify research findings that could be utilized in practice, and/or postulate additional reserach questions or hypotheses. Consult with a nurse researcher to help develop a research study. Encourage students to begin collecting articles that can support further investigation.

## NURSE HEALER REFLECTIONS

Encourage students to use the chapter reflective questions as a guide to journal entries for exploring, understanding, and validating presence and healing.

# Chapter 25

# Relationships

## CHAPTER OBJECTIVES

Refer to chapter for specific theoretical, clinical, and personal objectives. These will provide guidelines for the integration of objectives in class presentation, experiential sessions, and student homework assignments.

## CHAPTER OVERVIEW

Healthy relationships increase health and wholeness. Healthy relationships help us to understand at a deep level our interconnectedness with people, nature, and the universe. When we are in healthy relationships, we exhibit mutual love, sharing, and the ability to forgive ourselves and others. As nurses focus on family systems theory and relationship patterns, they can counsel and empower individuals more effectively in learning healing strategies within the context of relationships.

## PROCESS EXERCISE NO. 25

(15-minute opening experiential session using music and healing objects if desired.)

### Vision of Healing: Accepting Ourselves and Others

Wholeness and healing can exist only when we have meaningful relationships. The extent to which we are willing to accept ourselves determines the quality of relationships. A relationship is healing if it nurtures expression of feelings, needs, and desires and if it helps remove barriers to love.

Begin with a guided relaxation exercise (5 minutes) and gradually fade in music of choice. Suggest to students that they can close their eyes or leave their eyes open. Ask students who leave their eyes open to focus on a spot several feet in front of them. This allows for a greater ease in following the relaxation and imagery suggestions and reflective experience.

Using techniques for empowering relaxation and imagery scripts (see Chapters 21 and 22), gently weave into a guided imagery exercise the reflective questions from the Vision of Healing to increase awareness of current patterns in relationships and to identify relationships that are in need of healing. Pace these questions to allow time for images, emotions, and other responses. Bring closure to the imagery process.

With soft music still playing, invite students to record in a personal journal (3 to 5 minutes) any images, process questions and answers, or insight gained. Ask students to bring personal closure to this process. Gradually fade music out. Engage students in a gentle stretching exercise before the theory session begins.

## KEY CONCEPTS: THEORY AND RESEARCH

(1-hour presentation)

**OPTIONAL: GUEST SPEAKER(S) AND VIDEO(S)**

**Guest Speaker(s):** Invite one or more nurses who have a family counseling practice to discuss the dynamics of family counseling. Provide guest speaker(s) with the Instructor's Manual suggestions so the speaker(s) can become familiar with the students' assignment before class.

**Video(s):** Show a video of a practitioner describing and demonstrating one or more holistic modalities in family counseling (rent from media catalogue or purchase for school video library). Following the video presentation, ask students for their reactions and comments. Discuss the video and answer questions.

**Definitions:** Review definitions and incorporate into presentation.

**Patterns of Interactions and Relationships:** Discuss how effective awareness requires us to examine our daily interactions from three different perspectives of professional nursing practice.

**Effective Personal Characteristics that Build, Maintain, and Enhance Relationships:** Review the defenses that serve to protect an individual: denial, displacement, projection, rationalization, repression, and regression. Give examples of each.

Discuss the eight major personal characteristics that can assist us in moving toward effective relationships.

Review the work of the theorists in psychology who have further developed our understanding of effective relationship patterns. Name at least three.

## HOLISTIC CARING PROCESS

Focus on specifics of assessment, patterns/challenges/needs, outcomes, therapeutic care plan, implementation, and evaluation (Table 25-1 and Exhibit 25-1). Instruct students in the importance of developing their own style of preparation before, at the beginning of, during, and at the end of the session.

## EXPERIENTIAL EXERCISES

(2 hours. Incorporation of sharing circles and experiential exercises is encouraged for presentation. Refer to chapter section entitled "Specific Interventions" for details.)

**Counseling and Psychotherapy:** Review the common counseling strategies. Have students work in dyads. Ask students to discuss different clinical situations in which they have used several of the strategies listed. Share specific situations in which psychotherapy was indicated and the client was referred to a counselor, psychotherapist, and so on.

**Storytelling:** Review the guidelines that enhance the use of stories as therapy. Have students work in dyads. Have the first student tell a personal story and connect one story to the next. Then have the student that has been listening share the story themes that bridged from one story to the next. The listener should reflect on what part of the story was not being told with as much depth as other parts. Have students switch roles of sharing and listening.

**Development of Spiritual Understanding:** Encourage students to review the developmental process guidelines for gaining spiritual understanding. Next have students assess what strategies they currently use each day and what additional strategies would be helpful in deepening their spiritual understanding.

**Ways to Work through Fear:** Review the three levels of fear. Have students work in dyads and share a fear with each other. Ask students to identify the fear level that has been shared. After a student has shared a fear, the student that has been listening can read the five truths to help the student deal with the fear.

**Improved Communication:** Have students work in dyads. Direct the first student to access a stressful event in his or her life and also to access emotions of the event within the body (physiologic responses of heart beat, shallow breathing, cold hands, body tension, etc.) as the story is told. The student that is listening should observe any body language that reflects emotions. Discuss the results after each student tells a stressful event. Blood pressure cuffs, hand thermometers, or biofeedback equipment can be used before, during, and after the communication to demonstrate the dramatic and frequent changes in dialogue.

**Case Study:** Have students discuss case studies involving relationships as well as incorporate a case study into group presentation. Encourage students to share other client/patient stories and focus on the meaning of the stories, symptoms, illness and use of specific symbols and metaphors.

## DIRECTIONS FOR FUTURE RESEARCH

Have students choose one or more research questions as an area to explore; students should review the literature, identify research findings that could be utilized in practice, and/or postulate additional research questions or hypotheses. Consult with a nurse researcher to help develop a research study. Encourage students to begin collecting articles that can support further investigation.

## NURSE HEALER REFLECTIONS

Encourage students to use the chapter reflective questions as a guide to journal entries for exploring, understanding, and validating presence and healing.

# Chapter 26

# Dying in Peace

## CHAPTER OBJECTIVES

Refer to chapter for specific theoretical, clinical, and personal objectives. These will provide guidelines for the integration of objectives in class presentation, experiential sessions, and student homework assignments.

## CHAPTER OVERVIEW

Caring for and counseling a dying person and the family/significant others is an art. To die peacefully, to die with knowledge that life has had meaning and that one is connected through time and space to others, to God, and to the Universe, is to die well. Helping people to die well requires knowledge and skill as well as willingness to be intensively involved in the most intimate phases of another's life. Physical, spiritual, psychologic, and social distress must be addressed with concern and compassion. Theories of grief and loss, self-transcendence, myths and beliefs, and nearing-death awareness are particularly useful in formulating effective plans of care for the dying.

## PROCESS EXERCISE NO. 26

(15-minute opening experiential session using music and other healing objects if desired.)

### Vision of Healing: Releasing Attachment

Nothing in life prepares one for one's own death or the death of a loved one. True healing and dying in peace come from releasing one's attachment to the physical body and to the conflicting emotional and spiritual issues that hold one in bondage to this body and this world.

Begin with a guided relaxation exercise (5 minutes) and gradually fade in music of choice. Suggest to the students that they can close their eyes or leave their eyes open. Ask students who leave their eyes open to focus on a spot several feet in front of them. This allows for a greater ease in following the relaxation and imagery suggestions and reflective experience.

Using techniques for empowering relaxation and imagery scripts (see Chapters 21 and 22), gently weave into a guided relaxation and imagery exercise reflective scripts for dying in peace—Becoming Peaceful, Letting Go, Opening the Heart, and Forgiving Self and Others. Bring closure to the imagery process.

With soft music still playing, invite students to record in a personal journal (3 to 5 minutes) any images, process questions and answers or insight gained. Ask students to bring personal closure to this process. Gradually fade music out. Engage students in a gentle stretching exercise before the theory session begins.

## KEY CONCEPTS: THEORY AND RESEARCH

(1-hour presentation)

**OPTIONAL GUEST SPEAKER(S) AND VIDEO(S)**

**Guest Speaker(s):** Invite one or more hospice nurses to discuss holistic modalities that are used with individuals in various stages of death, dying, and grieving. Provide guest speaker(s) with the Instructor's Manual suggestions so the speaker(s) can become familiar with the students' assignment before class.

**Video(s):** Show a video about the dying or grieving process (rent from media catalogue or purchase for school video library). Following the video presentation, ask students for their reaction and comments. Discuss the video and answer questions.

**Definitions:** Review definitions and incorporate into presentation.

**Grief and Loss:** Explore grief theory in terms of the related concepts of loss, bereavement, and mourning.

**Self-Transcendence:** Examine the characteristics and qualities related to states of self-transcendence.

**Myths and Beliefs:** Explore how myths are our story lines, beliefs, and images. Discuss the five-stage program for creating empowering mythologies that will evoke courage and peace in dying.

**Nearing-Death Awareness:** Discuss the two categories of messages about death awareness from individuals in the dying process. Compare and contrast the similarities and differences in nearing-death awareness and near-death experiences.

## HOLISTIC CARING PROCESS

Focus on specifics of assessment, patterns/challenges/needs, outcomes, therapeutic care plan, implementation, and evaluation (Table 26–1 and exhibit 26–2). Instruct students in the importance of developing their own style off preparation before, at the beginning of, during, and at the end of the session.

## EXPERIENTIAL EXERCISES

(2 hours. Incorporation of sharing circles and experiential exercises is encouraged for class presentation. Refer to the chapter section entitled "Specific Interventions" for details.)

**Planning and Ideal Death:** Engage students in exploring the reflective questions about planning an ideal death. This process provides enormous insight about death, myths, beliefs, problem-solving, loving, and forgiving.

**Learning Forgiveness:** Have students review the steps to forgiving self and others. Next, provide time for students to write out or share with another student each of theses steps in forgiving self and forgiving another person.

**Relaxation and Imagery Scripts for Peace in Dying:** Provide time for students to experience each of the relaxation and imagery exercises and to share with each other their experiences. These exercises allow students to learn how to open and soften and how to be present in each daily moment, which leads to being in the moment with the death and dying process.

**The Pain Process:** Explore how the physical body may be experiencing pain but the mind's fear of pain is often more intense.

**Blending Breaths/Co-meditation:** Demonstrate the steps in co-meditation breathing.

Have students practice comeditation breathing in dyads. Following the experience, encourage students to share the co-meditation breathing experience.

**Mantras and Prayers:** Ask students to write or choose a mantra or special prayer. Invite students to share their mantras or prayers with the group. Have students share when they used prayer in their own lives as well as when they prayed for another or were told by friends or family that they were being prayed for or had been prayed for at certain times, such as during difficult situations.

**Reminiscing and Life Review:** Ask students to work in dyads and to guide each other using the life review process. Allow time for the sharing the experience.

**Leave-Taking Rituals:** Explore the importance of leave-taking rituals and different ways to work through the death of a loved one. Invite students to review certain rituals such as observing holidays, rearranging and giving away, letting grief be present, sustaining hope and faith, releasing anger and tears, healing memories, and getting unstuck. Invite the sharing of personal stories of working through grief.

**Case Study:** Have students discuss case studies involving death and grief counseling as well as incorporate a case study into group presentation. Encourage students to share other client/patient stories and to focus on the meaning of the stories, symptoms, illness, and use of specific symbols and metaphors.

## DIRECTIONS FOR FUTURE RESEARCH

Have students choose one or more research questions as an area to explore; students should review the literature, identify research findings that could be utilized in practice, and/or postulate additional research questions or hypotheses. Consult with a nurse researcher to help develop a research study. Encourage students to begin collecting articles that can support further investigation.

## NURSE HEALER REFLECTIONS

Encourage students to use the chapter reflective questions as a guide to journal entries for exploring, understanding, and validating presence and healing.

Chapter 27

# Weight Management Counseling

## CHAPTER OBEJECTIVES

Refer to chapter for specific theoretical, clinical, and personal objectives. These will provide guidelines for the integration of objectives in class presentation, experiential session, and student homework assignments.

## CHAPTER OVERVIEW

Obesity is a major health risk and is on the increase. The holistic self-care model is designed to assist overweight clients with individualized nutritional, exercise, and psychosocial-spiritual strategies for long-term pursuit of healthier and happier lifestyles.

## PROCESS EXERCISE NO. 27

(15-minute opening experiential session using music and at least one raisin per student.)

### Vision of Healing: Nourishing Wisdom

Often we eat in an unconscious manner. The following exercise is one of mindfulness and being present in the moment as we eat. Give each student a single raisin.

Begin with a guided relaxation exercise (5 minutes) and gradually fade in music of choice. Suggest to students that they can close their eyes or leave their eyes open. Ask students who leave their eyes open to focus on a spot several feet in front of them. This allows for a greater ease in following the relaxation and imagery suggestions and reflective experience.

Using techniques for empowering relaxation and imagery scripts (see Chapters 21 and 22), gently weave into a guided imagery exercise reflective questions about how the raisin feels in the mouth. As a guide, place a raisin in your mouth, allowing it just to be. As you experience the raisin taking different moves with increased salivation, as it goes from being shriveled to being plump, guide the students in maintaining focus on one raisin for 10 minutes or longer.

As the guide, recite the following: "Place a single raisin on your tongue and just let the raisin be. Do not bite or chew it. It will roll of your tongue and move around in your mouth with increased salivation. Just notice all the parts of your mouth that the raisin touches. After the raisin has swelled and is smooth (5–10 minutes) gently bite into it, noticing the juice, the meat, and the sweetness of the raisin. Notice the sensation of swallowing the single raisin. What images or memories come?" (This raisin exercise can take 10 minutes or longer.) Bring closure to the imagery process.

With soft music still playing invite students to record in a personal journal (3 to 5 minutes) any images, process questions and answers, or insight gained. ask students to bring personal closure to this process. Gradually fade music out. Engage students in a gentle stretching exercise before the theory session begins.

## KEY CONCEPTS: THEORY AND RESEARCH

(1 hour presentation)
**OPTIONAL: GUEST SPEAKER(S) AND VIDEO(S)**

**Guest Speaker(s):** Invite a nurse and/or nutritionist who focuses on nutrition education. Provide guest speaker(s) with the Instructor's Manual suggestions so the speaker(s) can become familiar with the students' assignment before class.

**Video(s):** Show a video of a practitioner describing and demonstrating one or more holistic modalities in regard to nutrition (rent from media catalogue or purchase for school video library). Following the video presentation, ask students for their reactions and comments. Discuss the video and answer questions.

**Definitions:** Review definitions and incorporate into presentation.

**Weigh Management Approaches:** Compare and contrast the biologic, behavioral, psychologic, and cognitive approaches to weight management.

**Failure of Traditional Weight Management Interventions:** Summarize the theoretical and research literature that explains why Americans have a growing weight problem.

**New Weight-Management Interventions:** Discuss cognitive restructuring based on reversal theory as a new weight management intervention.

**Holistic Self-Care Model:** Explore the nutritional, exercise, and psycho-social-spiritual strategies within the holistic self-care model for long-term weight management.

## HOLISTIC CARING PROCESS

Focus on specifics of assessment, patterns/challenges/needs, outcomes, therapeutic care plan, implementation, and evaluation (Table 27–1 and Exhibit 27–6). Instruct students in the importance of developing their own style of preparation before, at the beginning of, during, and at the end of the session.

## EXPERIENTIAL EXERCISES

(2 hours. Incorporation of sharing circles and experiential exercises is encouraged for class presentation. Refer to chapter section entitles "Specific Interventions" for details.)

**Stages of Change:** Ask students to identify the outcomes, nursing prescription, and methods of evaluation for each of the five stages of change.

**EAT for Hunger:** Invite students to explore the first cognitive restructuring nutritional strategy based on reversal theory, called "EAT" for hunger."

**Exercise for LIFE strategy:** Invite students to explore the steps in carrying out the "exercise for LIFE" strategy.

**STOP Emotional Eating:** Invite students to explore the steps involved in the "STOP emotional eating" strategy.

**Eight Ways of Being Human:** Ask students to experience the Ten-Minute Eight Ways of Being Human relaxation-affirmations exercise found in Exhibit 27–4.

**Case Study:** Have students discuss case studies involving weight management counseling as well as incorporate a case study into group presentation. Encourage students to share other client/patient stories and focus on the meaning of the stories, symptoms, illness, and use of specific symbols and metaphors.

## DIRECTIONS FOR FUTURE RESEARCH

Have students choose one or more research questions as an area to explore; students should review the literature, identify research findings that could be utilized in practice, and/or postulate additional research questions or hypotheses. Consult with a nurse researcher to help develop a research study. Encourage students to begin collecting articles that can support further investigation.

## NURSE HEALER REFLECTIONS

Encourage students to use the chapter reflective questions as a guide to journal entries for exploring, understanding, and validating presence and healing.

Chapter 28

# Smoking Cessation: Freedom from Risk

## CHAPTER OBJECTIVES

Refer to chapter for specific theoretical, clinical, and personal objectives. These will provide guidelines for the integration of objectives in class presentation, experiential sessions, and student homework assignments

## CHAPTER OVERVIEW

Becoming a successful ex-smoker requires commitment to change. For most individuals, smoking cessation is a step-by-step process. When preparation and healing rituals are incorporated into the change process, the individual has more success in sustaining smoking cessation. Smoking cessation programs must address behavioral and lifestyle changes.

## PROCESS EXERCISE NO. 28

(15-minute opening experiential session using music and healing objects if desired.)

### Vision of Healing: Acknowledging Fear

Fear of failure, fear of weight gain, and so on, are fears that smokers encounter as they begin the change toward becoming a nonsmoker. Have students experience ordinary fears that surface each day.

Begin with a guided relaxation exercise (5 minutes) and gradually fade in music of choice. Suggest to students that they can close their eyes or leave their eyes open. Ask students who leave their eyes open to focus on a spot several feet in front of them. This allows for a greater ease in following the relaxation and imagery suggestions and reflective experience.

Using techniques for empowering relaxation and imagery scripts (see Chapters 21 and 22), gently weave into a guided imagery exercise reflective questions about different fears such as fear of failure, rejection, the unknown, isolation, dying, loss of control, and so forth. Invite students to bring into their imagery process a specific fear and to reflect on the questions listed. Bring closure to the imagery process. With soft music still playing invite students to record in a personal journal (3 to 5 minutes) any images, process questions and answers, or insight gained. Ask students to bring personal closure to this process. Gradually fade music out. Engage students in a gentle stretching exercise before the theory session begins.

## KEY CONCEPTS: THEORY AND RESEARCH

(1-hour presentation)
**OPTIONAL: GUES SPEAKER(S) AND VIDEO(S)**

**Guest Speaker(s):** Invite one or more nurses who integrate holistic modalities into a smoking cessation program. Provide guest speaker(s) with the Instructor's Manual suggestions so the speaker(s) can become familiar with the students' assignments before class.

**Video(s):** Show a video of a practitioner describing and demonstrating one or more holistic modalities in regard to smoking cessation (rent from media catalogue or purchase for school video library). Following the video presentation, ask students for their reactions and comments. Discuss video and answer questions.

**Definitions:** Review definitions and incorporate into presentation.

**Prevalence of Smoking and Its Health Consequences:** Discuss the prevalence of smoking and its physiologic effects on the body.

**Strategies for Smoking Cessation:** Review research related to successful smoking cessation programs.

## HOLISTIC CARING PROCESS

Focus on specifics of assessment, patterns/challenges/needs, outcomes, therapeutic care plan, implementation, and evaluation (Table 28–2 and Exhibit 28–1). Instruct students in the importance of developing their own style of preparation before, at the beginning of, during, and at the end of the session.

## EXPERIENTAL EXERCISES

(2 hours. Incorporation of sharing circles and experiential exercises is encouraged for class presentation. Refer to chapter section entitled "Specific Interventions" for details.)

**Relaxation and Imagery Skills:** Explore active images, process images, and end-state images for smoking cessation.

**Recording of Habits:** Discuss how smoking is a pervasive, automatic habit. Most smokers need to keep a diary of when, where, and how often they smoke and what moods are associated with smoking. See reflective questions listed to help a client record data in a diary. If any students are smokers, have them assess where they are in the change process and the next steps to take toward becoming a successful nonsmoker.

**Preparation for Quit Date:** Reinforce the need for preparation for the quit date. The goal is to be a nonsmoker in 5 days.

**Preparation for Nicotine Withdrawal:** Discuss the three different strategies for coping with nicotine withdrawal.

**Smoke-Free Body and Environment:** Emphasize the strategies for body detoxification and cleaning of the living environment.

**Identification of Habit Breakers:** Review strategies for identifying when smoking is most likely to occur and creating habit breakers to replace negative smoking behaviors.

**Assertion of Bill of Rights:** Explore strategies to help smokers become aware of their right to be smoke free.

**Integration of Rewards:** Explore strategies to create rewards to help a smoker become a successful nonsmoker.

**Reinforcement of Positive Self-Talk:** Explore strategies to help smokers recognize how interconnected feelings, moods, behaviors, and motivation affect physiology.

**Smoking Cessation Imagery Scripts:** Integrate strategies for enhancing the imagery process for smoking cessation. Scripts include setting a quit date, cleansing the body and environment, recognizing signals for smoking, and incorporating nutritious eating and exercise.

**Case Study:** Have students discuss case studies involving smoking cessation counseling as well as incorporate a case study into group presentation. Encourage students to share other client/patient stories and focus on the meaning of the stories, symptoms, illness, and use of specific symbols and metaphors.

## DIRECTIONS FOR FUTURE RESEARCH

Have students choose one or more research questions as an area to explore; students should review the literature, identify research findings that could be utilized in practice, and/or postulate additional research questions or hypotheses. Consult with a nurse researcher to help develop a research study. Encourage students to begin collecting articles that can support further investigation.

## NURSE HEALER REFLECTIONS

Encourage students to use the chapter reflective questions as a guide to journal entries for exploring, understanding, and validating presence and healing.

Chapter 29

# Addiction and Recovery Counseling

## CHAPTER OBJECTIVES

Refer to chapter for specific theoretical, clinical, and personal objectives. These will provide guidelines for the integration of objectives in class presentation, experiential sessions and student homework assignments.

## CHAPTER OVERVIEW

Addiction is a disconnection from the human spirit in which a person develops a dependence on various aspects of the external world—a substance, a person, a situation, or a behavior. It often leads to a dysfunctional relationship in which the participants are codependent. The addicted individual must acknowledge that he or she is not alone in the struggle. To overcome an addiction, a person must first admit that the addiction exists. The best chance for recovery occurs when a person has the support of close friends and family, joins a support group, finds a sponsor, and learns new habits to change old behaviors.

## PROCESS EXERCISE NO. 29

(15-minute opening experiential session using music and other healing objects if desired.)

### Vision of Healing: Changing One's World View

Introduce students to the concept of world view and to the idea that at any given time an individual has a world view. A shift in the individual's world view is a fundamental and essential step to overcoming an addiction.

Begin with a guided relaxation exercise (5 minutes) and gradually fade in music of choice. Suggest to students that they can close their eyes or leave their eyes open. Ask the students who leave their eyes open to focus on a spot several feet in front of them. This allows for a greater ease in following the relaxation and imagery suggestions and reflective experience.

Using techniques for empowering relaxation and imagery scripts (see Chapter 21 and 22), gently weave into a guided imagery exercise reflective questions about world view and changing one's world view as given in the healing reflection. Into this script incorporate a world view about daily activities that can assist in caring for self and enhancing well-being. Bring closure to the imagery process.

With soft music still playing, invite students to record in a personal journal (3 to 5 minutes) any images, process. Gradually fade music out. Engage students in a gentle stretching exercise before the theory session begins.

## KEY CONCEPTS: THEORY AND RESEARCH

(1-hour presentation)

**OPTIONAL: GUEST SPEAKER(S) AND VIDEO(S)**

**Guest Speaker(s):** Invite one or more nurses who integrate holistic modalities in an addiction counseling practice. Provide guest speaker(s) with the Instructor's Manual suggestions so the speaker(s) can become familiar with the student's assignment before class.

**Video(s):** Show a video of a practitioner describing and demonstrating one or more holistic modalities in a substance abuse program (rent from media catalogue or purchase for school video library). Following the video presentation, ask students for their reactions and comments. Discuss the video and answer questions.

**Definitions:** Review definitions and incorporate into presentation.

**Prevalence of Alcoholic and Social Drinkers:** Discuss prevalence, death rates, cost, and theories of alcoholism.

**Defining Addictions:** According to Alcoholics Anonymous, alcoholism is "a mental obsession and a physical compulsion." Discuss the patterns and behaviors that are recognizable as addictive processes.

**The Cycle of Addiction:** Discuss the cycle of addiction and the addictive feelings and physical signs.

**Stages of the Addictive Cycle:** Examine the early, middle, and late stages of addictive behavior.

**Models of Addiction:** Explore the different models of addiction: genetic disease model, dysfunctional family system model, self-medication model, psychosexual psychoanalytic model, ego psychology model, cultural model, character defect model of Alcoholics Anonymous, trance model, transpersonal-intoxication model, and transpersonal-existential model.

**The Vulnerability Model of Recovery:** Discuss the holistic nursing model of the recovery process that considers the biologic, emotional, social, familial, neurochemical, and spiritual aspects of addiction (Exhibit 29–1).

Discuss primary prevention of addiction. Examine early education as a key intervention in preventing substance abuse. Include in the discussion the key obstacle to entering into the healing process of recovery and the descriptions and definitions of denial (Exhibit 29–2).

Address the importance of detoxification. Introduce the 12 steps of Alcoholics Anonymous (Exhibit 29–3). Explore enabling, assistance to strengthen early recovery, nutritional issues in early alcoholism recovery, bodywork and energy work in early recovery, and relapse.

Address the holistic approach to tertiary prevention to deepen the recovery process. Integrate the spectrum of willfulness (Figure 29–1), the spectrum of will-lessness (Figure 29–2), and the spectrum of willingness (Figure 29–3).

Explore spiritual development and transformation, and bodymind responses in the recovery process.

## HOLISTIC CARING PROCESS

Focus on specifics of assessment, patterns/challenges/needs, outcomes, therapeutic care plan, implementation, and evaluation for addiction and recovery counseling (Table 29–1). Instruct students in the importance of developing their own style of preparation before, at the beginning of, during, and at the end of the session.

## EXPERIENTIAL EXERCISES

(2 hours. Incorporation of sharing circles and experiential exercises is encouraged in class presentation. Refer to the chapter section entitled "Specific Interventions" for details.)

**Are You a Problem Drinker?** Encourage students to complete this important self-assessment (Exhibit 29–4). If students are concerned about a friend or family member who may have an addiction, this tool may be used.

**Support from Family and Friends:** Encourage students to interview a person who has been part of a family intervention team to become more aware of the detailed planning necessary for a successful intervention.

**Support Groups and Professional Help:** Encourage students to attend a meeting of a 12-step program for breaking addictions and to discuss with each other their personal responses to attending a support meeting. Reinforce the importance of addressing colleague addictions in the workplace and discuss ways to be part of a support intervention team.

**Learning to Tell a Personal Story:** Have students discuss recurrent story themes in 12-step program meetings and the ways in which addicted individuals release their attachments to substances, people, situations, or behaviors.

**Resistance to Spirituality:** Have students identify any spiritual resistance or discomfort that is personally experienced when phrases or terms such as "in relationship to God," "Higher Power," and so on, are used to assist in breaking addictions.

**Relaxation and Imagery:** Explore how relaxation and imagery skills are strategies to assist the addicted person to access feelings, behaviors, and emotions, and to learn how to sustain new health behaviors.

**Healing Addictions Imagery Scripts:** Guide students with scripts that incorporate strategies for enhancing relaxation and the imagery process of being addiction free. Scripts include affirming strengths, overcoming drink/drug signals, rehearsing Alcoholics Anonymous meetings, learning to trust and forgive, and replacing old patterns.

**Case Study:** Have students discuss case studies involving addiction and recovery counseling as well as incorporate a case study into group presentation. Encourage students to share other patient stories and to focus on the meaning of the symptoms, disease, illness, and use of specific symbols and metaphors.

## DIRECTIONS FOR FUTURE RESEARCH

Have students choose one or more research questions as an area to explore; students should review the literature, identify research findings that could be utilized in practice, and/or postulate additional research questions or hypotheses. Consult with a nurse researcher to help develop a research study. Encourage students to begin collecting articles that can support further investigation.

## NURSE HEALER REFLECTIONS

Encourage students to use the chapter reflective questions as a guide to journal entries for exploring, understanding, and validating presence and healing.

Chapter 30

# Incest and Child Sexual Abuse

## CHAPTER OBJECTIVES

Refer to chapter for specific theoretical, clinical, and personal objectives. These will provide guidelines for the integration of objectives in class presentation, experiential sessions, and student homework assignments.

## CHAPTER OVERVIEW

Working with survivors of abuse or violence is one of the most difficult experiences, but it is also one of the most rewarding. Because of a reluctance to inquire, one can work with a client over a long period of time without knowing that he or she has been or perhaps even still is involved in a violent situation.

## PROCESS EXERCISE NO. 30

(15-minute opening experiential session using music and healing objects if desired.)

### Vision of Healing: Recovering the Self and Maintaining the Self

The recovery of the self moves in cycles and layers. Both client and nurse must be prepared for this circuitous journey to wholeness, taking each new stage as reassurance of progress.

Begin with a guided relaxation exercise (5 minutes) and gradually fade in music of choice. Suggest to students that they can close their eyes or leave their eyes open. Ask students who leave their eyes open to focus on a spot several feet in front of them. This allows for a greater ease in following the relaxation and imagery suggestions and reflective experience.

Using techniques for empowering relaxation and imagery scripts (see Chapters 21 and 22), gently weave reflective questions into a guided imagery exercise, using an artichoke as a metaphor of the self. To get to the heart of the artichoke, we must peel away layer after layer. To get to our own hearts, we must delve below the outer surface to discover our essential core of healing.

Invite students to begin to peel away the outer layer of burdens and problems, and to begin to go below the surface, deep into the self, to find the inner healing resources present within the moment to bring about healing. In the imagination, have students complete the following sentence: "The part of me that is most in need of healing in this moment is. . . . The thing that I can do in this moment to bring about the healing is. . . ." Bring closure to the imagery process.

With soft music still playing, invite students to record in a personal journal (3 to 5 minutes) any images, process questions and answers, or insight gained. Ask students to bring personal closure to this process. Gradually fade music out. Engage students in a gentle stretching exercise before the theory session begins.

## KEY CONCEPTS: THEORY AND RESEARCH

(1-hour presentation)

OPTIONAL: GUEST SPEAKER(S) AND VIDEO(S)

**Guest Speaker(s):** Ask one or more sexual abuse counselors to address precautions when working with survivors, bodymind responses, and the process of moving through memories. Provide guest speaker(s) with the Instructor's Manual suggestions so the speaker(s) can become familiar with the students' assignment before class.

**Video(s):** Review a video that explores the dynamics of using holistic modalities in sexual abuse counseling (rent from media catalogue or purchase for school video library). Following the video presentation, ask students for their reactions and comments. Discuss the video and answer questions.

**Definitions:** Review definitions and incorporate into presentation.

**History of Incest and Child Sexual Abuse:** Explore the long, multicultural, multicontinent history of child sexual abuse. Discuss current issues and theories as documented in the literature.

**Emotional, Behavioral, and Physical Consequences of Incest and Child Sexual Abuse:** Review and discuss the long-term ramifications of abuse in early life. List some of the general physical symptoms.

## HOLISTIC CARING PROCESS

Focus on specifics of assessment, patterns/challenges/needs, outcomes, therapeutic care plan, implementation, and evaluation (Table 30–1 and Exhibit 30–1). Instruct students in the importance of developing their own style of preparation before, at the beginning of, during, and at the end of the session.

## EXPERIENTIAL EXERCISES

(2 hours. Incorporation of sharing circles and experiential exercises is encouraged in class presentation. Refer to chapter section entitled "Specific Interventions" for details.)

**Grounding Skills:** Explore the dissociation that may occur with painful memories and the way in which dissociation may prevent survivors from recognizing dangerous situations, making them more vulnerable to further victimization. Have students share different grounding strategies to use for self or others to stay present rather than becoming overwhelmed by memories.

**Relaxation:** Examine how disturbing flashbacks and body memories may surface when the physical armor of tension is quieted. Explore how individuals may equate relaxation with vulnerability that conflicts with their hypervigilance. Discuss the best relaxation strategies for abuse survivors.

**Imagery:** Explore how imagery can be used as a healing modality to assist the abuse survivor in connecting with the suppressed emotions surrounding the abuse experience as well as in coming face to face with the perpetrator in the imagination. Review the imagery process steps discussed in the text of acting "as if"; that is, of having the client get in touch with the somatic response and be face to face with the perpetrator. As the client rehearses this event in safe, structured environment, an opportunity is created for the person to move beyond the pain, anger, and sadness of the situation.

**Biofeedback:** Examine biofeedback as a strategy for helping abuse survivors connect with body sensations and gain control over uncomfortable physiologic responses. Discuss the precautions when working with different types of abuse survivors.

**Hypnosis and Self-Hypnosis:** Explore how hypnosis and self-hypnosis are structured processes of relaxation designed to produce a state of dissociation that helps an individual to get in touch with unconscious parts of the self, such as feelings, memories, or awareness.

**Bodywork:** Explore how bodywork is a means of abuse survivors to learn to reconnect to their body responses, a path to the retrieval of memories, and a way of speeding the retrieval of memories and the recovery of body sensations.

**Writing:** Encourage students to prepare a family record and note the presence of any perpetrators or victims of violence or members with substance abuse or eating disorders. If painful memories or associations occur for any of the students, encourage them to learn healing strategies and to seek out assistance and resolution of painful memories with a nurse therapist or to join a support group that is under the guidance of a trained counselor.

**Art Therapy:** Review the work of art therapists or sexual abuse counselors who have used art, collages, photography, clay, masks, and so on, to tap into deep feelings and understanding that are inaccessible to the verbal realm alone. Discuss recurring themes, symbols, colors, or objects that give personal clues to memory fragments or thoughts that are not yet safe to put into words.

**Video Therapy:** Review or develop policies and procedures for dealing with the emotional and physical needs of victims of abuse in emergency situations or other clinical situations. Discuss the five-stage process of video disclosure.

**Anger Expression and Management:** Have students work in groups of three to five people and share their personal style of anger management that allows expression of anger without injury to self or others.

**Case Study:** Have students discuss case studies involving sexual abuse counseling as well as incorporate a case study into group presentation. Encourage students to share other client/patient stories and to focus on the meaning of symptoms, disease, illness, and use of specific symbols and metaphors.

## DIRECTIONS FOR FUTURE RESEARCH

Have students choose one or more research questions as an area to explore; students should review the literature, identify research findings that could be utilized in practice, and/or postulate additional research questions or hypotheses. Consult with a nurse researcher to help develop a research study. Encourage students to begin collecting articles that can support further investigation.

## NURSE HEALER REFLECTIONS

Encourage students to use the chapter reflective questions as a guide to journal entries for exploring, understanding, and validating presence and healing.

# Chapter 31

# Aromatherapy

## CHAPTER OBJECTIVES

Refer to chapter for specific theoretical, clinical, and personal objectives. These will provide guidelines for the integration of objectives in class presentation, experiential sessions, and student homework assignments.

## CHAPTER OVERVIEW

Aromatherapy is an ancient therapy that began a modern renaissance in the 1940s. This therapy utilizes essential oils obtained by steam distillation from aromatic plants for the physical, psychological, and spiritual benefit of the recipient. Any one of a great variety of chemical components travel via the nose to the olfactory bulb where trigger responses in the limbic system of the brain occur. Essential oils are thought to work at psychological, physiological, and cellular levels. The effects of aroma can be relaxing or stimulating depending on one's previous experience. There are a number of endorsed aromatherapy courses for nurses who wish to use this therapy with clients.

## PROCESS EXERCISE NO. 31

(15-minute opening experiential session using music and healing objects if desired.)

### Vision of Healing: Healing through the Senses

Aromatherapy uses essential oils to awaken the senses. Sometimes the therapy is used to stimulate and refresh while othertimes it is used to soothe and relax. A skilled therapist makes judgements for the client based on interview and observation and selects the most appropriate oil for the right occasion. When used with skill, aromatherapy can create a general feeling of well-being that can permeate all of our activities and that enables quicker thinking, allows for more restful sleep, and facilitates relaxation that leads to a deeper spiritual understanding.

Begin with a guided relaxation exercise (5 minutes) and gradually fade in music of choice. Suggest to students that they can close their eyes or leave their eyes open. If eyes are left open ask them to find a spot several feet in front of them to focus on. This allows for a greater ease in following the relaxation and imagery suggestions and reflective experience.

Using techniques for empowering relaxation and imagery scripts (see Chapters 21 and 22), gently weave into a guided imagery exercise the following reflective questions. What does aromatherapy mean to you? How do you feel when you smell the odor of an American Beauty Rose? How do you feel when you smell the odor of baking bread? Add three to five more reflective questions in regard to smell. Bring closure to the imagery process.

With soft music still playing, invite students to record in a personal journal (3 to 5 minutes) any images, process questions and answers, or insight gained. Ask students to bring personal closure to this process. Gradually fade music out. Engage students in a gentle stretching exercise before the theory session ends.

## KEY CONCEPTS: THEORY AND RESEARCH

(1-hour presentation)
**OPTIONAL: GUEST SPEAKER(S) AND VIDEO(S)**

**Guest Speaker(s):** Invite a nurse who integrates holistic modalities, specifically aromatherapy in her/his practice. Provide guest speaker(s) with the Instructor's Manual suggestions so the speaker(s) can become familiar with the students' reading assignment before class.

**Video:** Show a video of a practitioner who describes, demonstrates, and integrates one or more touch modalities (rent from medical catalogue or purchase for school video library). Following the video presentation, ask students for their reactions and comments. Discuss the video and answer questions.

**Definitions:** Review definitions and incorporate into presentation.

**Aromatherapy in Ancient Times:** Review the history of aromatherapy. Discuss the multi-thousand-year use of distilled oils from herbs and how many, varied cultures used this therapy. Discuss the modern renaissance that began in France just prior to World War II.

**Touch in Aromatherapy:** Aromatherapy is often used with a gentle stroking sequence of movements call the 'm' technique. This registered method of touch is suitable when massage is inappropriate either because the recipient is too fragile or the giver is not trained in massage. Gentle friction enhances absorption of essential oils through the skin into the blood stream.

**Olfaction:** The fastest effects from aromatherapy are through olfaction. Discuss the chemical components and the pathways to the brain with the ensuing effect on the limbic system.

**Administration and Techniques:** Explore and discuss the various ways to use aromatherapy via the senses of smell through inhalation and topically via touch. The oils can be used either by a trained professional or via self-administration.

## HOLISTIC CARING PROCESS

Focus on specifics of assessment, pattern/challenges/needs, outcomes, therapeutic care plan, implementation, and evaluation. Instruct students in the importance of developing their own style of preparation before, at the beginning of, during, and at the end of the session.

## EXPERIENTIAL EXERCISES

(2 hours. Incorporation of sharing circles and experiential exercises is encouraged in class presentations.)

**Awareness:** Direct students to spend some time in focused concentration to increase awareness of their olfactory senses. Bring strong smelling items to class to stimulate the students to consider this modality (i.e., garlic, perfume, fresh fruit, herbs, shoe polish, and other self-scented items). Have students close their eyes, then smell, identify, and discuss sensations and feelings generated by the odor.

**Touch and aromatherapy:** Follow the above exercise, but incorporate the sensation of touch simultaneously. For example, stroke a fresh, flowering lavender stalk across the face or forearm and ask the student to describe the sensation and its meaning to him/her.

**Case Study:** Have students discuss case studies as well as incorporate a case study into group presentation. Encourage students to share other client/patient stories and to focus on the meaning of the symptoms, disease, illness, and use of specific symbols and metaphors.

## DIRECTIONS FOR FUTURE RESEARCH

Have students choose one or more research questions as an area to explore; students should review the literature, identify research findings that could be utilized in practice, and/or postulate additional research questions or hypotheses. Consult with a nurse researcher to help develop a research study. Encourage students to begin collecting articles that can support further investigation.

## NURSE HEALER REFLECTIONS

Encourage students to use the chapter reflective questions as a guide to journal entries for exploring, understanding, and validating presence and healing.

# Chapter 32

# Relationship-Centered Care and Healing Initiative in a Community Hospital

## CHAPTER OBJECTIVES

Refer to chapter for specific theoretical, clinical, and personal objectives. These will provide guidelines for the integration of objectives in class presentation, experiential session, and student homework assignments.

## CHAPTER OVERVIEW

The Healing Health Care Philosophy at St. Charles Medical Center (SCMC), Bend, Oregon, has created a prototype that demonstrates how every concept and intervention contained within this book can be integrated into practice, education, and research. Our challenge is to follow their lead and know that healing health care is a reality.

## PROCESS EXERCISE NO.32

(15-minute opening experiential session using music and healing objects if desired.)

### Vision of Healing: Nursing Voices of St. Charles Medical Center

As we explore nursing voices/stories related to healing health care, we are able to access those events that are most important as well as more easily identify what it means to be in the service of healing health care. As we reflect on our personal experience with daily events, we move closer to a deeper understanding of holism.

Begin with a guided relaxation exercise (5 minutes) and gradually fade in music of choice. Suggest to students that they can close their eyes or leave their eyes open. If eyes are left open ask them to find a spot several feet in front of them to focus on. This allows for a greater ease in following the relaxation and imagery suggestions and reflective experience.

Ask for seven participants in the class to each read out loud to the other students one of the seven short voices/stories listed in the Vision of Healing that were written by SCMC nurses.

With soft music still playing, invite students to record in a personal journal (3 to 5 minutes) any images, process questions and answers, or insight gained. Ask students to bring personal closure to this process. Gradually fade music out. Engage students in a gentle stretching exercise before the theory session begins.

## KEY CONCEPTS: THEORY AND RESEARCH

(1- hour presentation)
**OPTIONAL: GUEST SPEAKER(S) AND VIDEO(S)**

**Guest Speaker(s):** Invite a nurse who integrates holistic modalities in clinical practice or a panel of nurses in different practice settings that are guided in practice by a bio-psycho-social-spiritual model. Provide guest speaker(s) with the Instructor's Manual suggestions to become familiar with the student's reading assignment before class.

**Video:** Show a video of a practitioner describing and demonstrating one or more holistic modalities (rent from media catalog or purchase for school video library). Following the video presentation ask students for their reaction and comments. Discuss video and answer questions.

**Definitions:** Review definitions and incorporate into presentation.

**Healing Health Care Philosophy:** Provide an overview of the Healing Health Care Philosophy at St. Charles Medical Center (SCMC).

**About St. Charles Medical Center: Why and How a Healing Philosophy Became Integrated into the Hospital's Strategic Initiatives.** Review the steps in how SCMC was able to integrate a healing philosophy throughout the entire system that engaged all departments and all employees.

**Healing Ourselves and Our Relationships:** Explore the personal growth and development workshops at SCMC.

**Patient-Focused and Family-Focused Care:** Discuss the concepts of patient-focused and family-focused care, The Caring Model™ (Exhibit 32–1), Therapeutic Presence Core Competency (Exhibit 32–2), and RN/LPN Nursing Care Delivery Skills-Pain/Anxiety Management (Exhibit 32–3).

**Life Skills:** Explore the Center for Health and Learning (CHL), the New Direction Program, and Health Coaching Services (Exhibit 32–4).

**Life-Death Transition:** Discuss the SCMC Comfort Care Services, Comfort Care Patient Checklist (Exhibit 32–5), Satisfaction of Improved End-of-Life Survey (Figure 32–3), and the Deschutes County Coalition for Quality-End-Of-Life Care.

**Healing Has Many Dimensions:** Review the many dimensions and qualities contained within healing that include both the internal environment of a person and the external environment of the physical space (See Figure 32–1 to Figure 32–14).

**Arts in the Hospital:** Explore how art and music in a hospital environment are ways of caring for the soul.

**Healing Our Community:** Investigate how a hospital can partner with a community to increase the healing and health quality of both.

**Principle-Based Care Model:** Review professional nursing practice principles (See Exhibit 32–6) and the Health Management Model (Figure 32–12).

## EXPERIENTIAL EXERCISES

(2 hours. Incorporation of experiential exercises is encouraged for class presentation.)

**Integrating a Healing Health Care Philosophy and Model:** Using SCMC as a prototype, have students work in teams of 6 to 8 and assess their current work situation. Encourage them to role-play and imagine that they have been selected to be the visioning teams that are assigned to making changes in their workplace toward the SCMC prototype and model. Encourage them to be aware that they are the future leaders that will be implementing these new models of health and healing in hospitals and in communities, and will be taking it to a new level.

## DIRECTIONS FOR FUTURE RESEARCH

Have students choose one or more research questions as an area to explore; students should review the literature, identify research findings that could be utilized in practice, and/or postulate additional research questions or hypotheses. Consult with a nurse researcher to help develop a research study. Encourage students to begin collecting articles that can support further investigation.

**Nurse Healer Reflections:** Encourage students to use the chapter reflective questions as a guide to journal entries of exploring, understanding, and validating presence and healing.

Chapter 33

# Exploring Integrative Medicine and the Healing Environment: The Story of a Large Urban Acute Care Hospital

## CHAPTER OBJECTIVES

Refer to chapter for specific theoretical, clinical, and personal objectives. These will provide guidelines for the integration of objectives in class presentation, experiential session, and student homework assignments.

## CHAPTER OVERVIEW

A "Total Healing Environment" within Abbott Northwestern Hospital, Minneapolis, Minnesota, a large urban acute care hospital encompasses many elements. Although in the broad view it may seem to be an overwhelming accomplishment to achieve, the foundation is simple—relationships.

Whether we speak about the internal or external elements, the physical or psychological elements, it is all based on the interconnectedness of relationships. The dynamics of changing a culture is continuous and requires an openness to honor both the successes and the perceived failures. One strategic initiative in stimulating the hospital's changing culture is the development of integrative medicine.

## PROCESS EXERCISE NO. 33

(15-minute opening experiential session using music and healing objects if desired.)

### Vision of Healing: Transformation of the Acute Health Care Environment

As we explore nursing voices/stories related to healing health care, we are able to access those events that are most important as well as more easily identify what it means to be in the service of healing health care. As we reflect on our personal experience with daily events, we move closer to a deeper understanding of holism.

Ask a participant to read out loud "A Story of Healing" in the Vision of Healing. After this reading, invite all participants to respond to how they felt when they heard the story. Form triads and have students share moments of healing when they remember being there for another person, such as with a patient, a family member, or a friend. Explore what it felt like to be listened to in this way.

With soft music still playing, invite students to record in a personal journal (3-5 minutes) any images, process questions and answers, or insight gained. Ask students to bring personal closure to this process. Gradually fade music out. Engage students in a gentle stretching exercise before the theory session begins.

## KEY CONCEPTS: THEORY AND RESEARCH

(1-hour presentation)
**OPTIONAL: GUEST SPEAKER(S) AND VIDEO(S)**

**Guest Speaker(s):** Invite a nurse who integrates holistic modalities in clinical practice or a panel of nurses in different practice settings that are guided in practice by a bio-psycho-social-spiritual model. Provide guest speaker(s) with the Instructor's Manual suggestions to become familiar with the student's reading assignment before class.

**Video(s):** Show a video of a practitioner describing and demonstrating one or more holistic modalities (rent from media catalogue or purchase for school video library). Following the video presentation, ask students for their reaction and comments. Discuss video and answer questions.

**Definitions:** Review definitions and incorporate into presentation.

**Total Healing Environment Model: Large Urban Acute Care Hospital:** Review the framework and the four components of the "Total Healing Environment" at Abbott Northwestern Hospital, Minneapolis, Minnesota.

**Healing Environment Assessment:** Discuss the purpose and findings of the Healing Environment Survey, the chart audit, department team assessments, and the patient admission survey.

**Analysis of the Healing Environment Assessment:** Explore the data collected from the four assessments and how it provided the framework for the strategic plan.

**Initiating the Culture Change:** Review the three components of the holistic philosophy that were introduce to the staff: relationship-centered care, presence and intention, and psychoneuroimmunology.

**Integrative Medicine:** Discuss integrative medicine, and the distinctions of integrative medicine complementary therapies, and alternative therapies. Explore integrative medicine at Abbott Northwestern Hospital, and the integrative medicine team, integrative medicine components, integrative medicine program principles, and functions of integrative medicine.

## EXPERIENTIAL EXERCISES

(2 hours. Incorporation of experiential exercises is encouraged for class presentation.)

**Total Healing Environment Model: Large Urban Acute Care Hospital:** Using Abbott Northwestern as a prototype, have students work in teams of 6 to 8 and assess their current work situation. Encourage them to role-play and imagine that they have been selected to be the visioning teams that are assigned to making changes in their workplace toward the total healing environment prototype and model. Encourage them to be aware that they are the future leaders that will be implementing these new models of health and healing in hospitals and in communities, and will be taking it to new level.

## DIRECTIONS FOR FUTURE RESEARCH

Have students choose one or more research questions as an area to explore; students should review the literature, identify research findings that could be utilized in practice, and/or postulate additional research questions or hypotheses. Consult with a nurse researcher to help develop a research study. Encourage students to begin collecting articles that can support further investigation.

## NURSE HEALER REFLECTIONS

Encourage students to use the chapter reflective questions as a guide to journal entries for exploring, understanding, and validating presence and healing.

## Appendix A

# Guidelines for Creating a Healing Tapestry

There are many unique learning opportunities and modalities for students and even practicing nurses to deepen their understanding of presence and healing. We have adapted the American Town Hall Wall* concept and call the process/experiential exercise "Creating a Healing Tapestry." The size of the healing tapestry is determined by class size. You can create several small or several large blank tapestries depending on preference. The blank tapestry can be a simple assemblage of large pieces of brown wrapping paper, or it can be a small or large blanket to which pieces of paper can be taped or pinned. However, we encourage that a special blank tapestry be created. Felt, for instance, is an ideal material for this use.

A tapestry created for use with 48 students is shown in Figure 4. The tapestry background is made of light purple felt and is framed with a 3″ black felt border. It is divided into forty-eight 8-1/2″ by 11″ squares, which are separated by 2″ black felt strips.

The 88″ × 82″ dimensions of the finished tapestry, which accommodate eight squares across and five squares down, was arrived at as follows:

| | |
|---|---|
| 68″ (8 × 8-1/2″ squares across) | 66″ (6 × 11″ squares down) |
| 6″ (2 × 2″ black felt side borders) | 6″ (2 × 3″ black felt bottom/top borders) |
| 14″ (7 × 2″ black felt dividing strips) | 10″ (5 × 2″ black felt dividing strips) |
| 88″ across the top of the tapestry | 82″ from top to bottom of the tapestry |

Felt comes in a variety of widths, all smaller than the dimensions required for the background. At least one seam will be required to attach two strips of the felt, which can then be cut to the 88″ × 82″ size.

Students can be given standard-size (8-1/2″ × 11″), light-colored construction paper and large black felt-tip markers, pens, and/or crayons with which to create their statements/expressions/drawings. A more elaborate exercise is for each student to select a small square of felt and create a pattern using a variety of colored yarns that are attached to the felt with glue. Students' paper or felt squares can be affixed to the tapestry by attaching adhesive-backed male Velcro dots to the back of the square, which will then easily adhere to a blank square on the felt tapestry.

It might be a good idea to create a number of statements/expressions/drawings of your own to add to blank paper squares, or to design yarn patterns on felt squares to complete the tapestry should you have slightly less student squares than appropriate for a finished tapestry.

Introduce students to the healing process as follows with music softly playing:

> Healing is a lifelong journey into understanding the wholeness of human existence. Along this journey, our lives mesh with those of clients, families, and colleagues, and moments of new meaning and insight emerge in the midst of crisis. Healing occurs when we help clients, families, others, and ourselves to embrace what is feared most. It occurs when we seek harmony and balance. Healing is learning how to open what has been closed so that we can expand our inner potentials. It is the fullest expression of ourselves that is demonstrated by the light and shadow and the male and female principles that reside within each of us. It is accessing what we have forgotten about connections, unity, and interdependence. With a new awareness of these inter-

relationships, healing becomes possible, and the experience of a nurse healer becomes actualized. A nurse healer is one who facilitates another person's growth toward wholeness (body-mind-spirit) or who assists another with stabilization of a disease process, recovery from illness, or transition to peaceful death.

Next, invite students to write different qualities of healing and healing moments, symbols, and so on, on colored construction paper or to create a small healing tapestry with felt and yarns. In a quiet, reflective manner, as music continues to play softly, ask students to attach their contributions to the blank tapestry, thus completing the healing tapestry. Allow time for group sharing.

There are many adaptations to this experience. Invite students to think of different word combinations as follows:

**Joy:** Invite joy, embrace joy, live joy, dance with joy, see joy in a cloud, share joy, embody joy.

**Wisdom:** See that you are wise, cherish wisdom, speak the truth, be fully present, listen with the heart, forgive ignorance, spread the light.

**Loving-kindness:** Trust love, let go of fear, let go of despair, love life, let go of anger, love the sacred, love who you are.

**Healing:** Heal thyself, heal family, heal the earth, heal with forgiveness, heal with love, heal with laughter, heal with faith.

*The authors wish to thank Beverly Dunaway and Sustainable Strategies, Mountain View, Arkansas, for the introduction to the American Town Hall Wall and assistance with photographs.

Appendix B

# Script: Creating a Healing Tapestry

INTRODUCTION: A tapestry of healing allows us to reflect on the dynamics of healing. Each of you will create a small tapestry that will be placed with other creations onto the blank tapestry. There is no right or wrong way. Just allow images to come during a guided relaxation and imagery experience.

DIRECTIONS: The following is written as if students will be applying colored yarns to a small colored square of felt. Colored construction paper, crayons, or colored markers may also be used. To affix the student's piece to the tapestry, a small adhesive-backed male Velcro dot will be attached to the back of the felt square after completion. Invite students to find a comfortable place to sit or lie down as the guided relaxation and imagery exercise begins; use music playing softly to enhance the process prior to the actual creating of their piece.

SCRIPT: As your mind becomes clearer and clearer, feel it becoming more and more alert. Somewhere deep inside of you, a light begins to glow. Sense this happening . . . the light growing brighter and more intense. . . . . This is your body-mind-spirit communication center. Breathe into it . . . energize it with your breath. The light is powerful and penetrating . . . and a beam begins to grow out of it to guide you in creating your small unique tapestry that will become part of a large group healing tapestry.

Imagine that you are beginning a small tapestry to contribute to a group healing tapestry. Create a healing space where you will do your sacred work. Right now, focus on your beautiful blank felt that will become part of the group tapestry . . . and the colors that appeal to the artist who resides within you.

In front of you are exquisite threads of many colors and textures, and shimmering metallics. . . . Choose the threads to represent your healing . . . a beautiful thread to represent each of your healing potentials . . . your joy, peace, harmony, kindness, presence . . . your courage, truth, patience . . . your love, honor, trust . . . your fears, strengths, weaknesses . . . your light and shadow . . . your clarity, humor, abundance . . . your memories, magical places, compassion, forgiveness . . . your wisdom, purpose, meaning. . . .

Select additional threads to represent releasing, opening, seeking, touching, caring, remembering, expressing, responding . . . more threads for affirming, changing, creating, intending . . . for sensing, planning, quieting, attuning . . . threads for softening, forgiving, clearing . . . for awakening, journeying, transcending, attending . . . threads for receiving, presencing, listening, doing . . . for being, enlivening, engaging . . . for letting go, entering the void. . . .

More threads represent healing of family, friends, colleagues . . . for community, global nations, and relations . . . for all things living and nonliving . . . for healing moments, hurting moments . . . spinning your healing threads of light from your healing core . . . your healing source of beingness. . . .

And now you are beginning to join each thread with your intrinsic rhythm. . . . Sit for a while . . . with rhythmic breathing. . . . Let the designs, colors, and movements of a spirit-filled tapestry begin to form. . . . And let your rhythms of healing spirit begin to dance. You are aware of becoming at one with the work, serving the work and the moment . . . feeling the energy of many high beings surrounding you . . . your soul expanding upward and outward . . . penetrating all of your energy systems . . . acknowledging what part of you is in need of healing . . . honoring the challenges before you . . . asking for new understanding in this healing process . . . receiving the inner wisdom . . . and new ways to connect with your higher self. . . .

If it seems right . . . choose some healing objects to incorporate into your tapestry. As you choose these objects, let the sacredness of each object speak to you . . . such as stones, flowers, seashells, medallions, beads, grasses . . . representing you, people, and things that are sacred . . . those who may be in need of remembrance or in need of healing.

Focusing now on the patterns and designs . . . the squares, circles, mosaics, or other images . . . that will flow into your healing tapestry. The time has come to begin the next phase. . . .

You feel the energy rising forth to begin the intermeshing, connecting, and coming together of the beautiful threads. . . . Begin now to push and pull with the rhythm of creating . . . adding sacred objects . . . breathing and feeling your intrinsic balance . . . journeying deep into your soul . . . tapping your inner wisdom, knowledge, and answers. . . .

You are now placing the final threads into the tapestry . . . feeling the energy . . . placing the final sacred objects in and on the tapestry. . . . The work has reached a stopping point for now. . . .

The energy fields . . . the weaving technology . . . your mind . . . your spirit . . . embracing the dynamic dance of flowing . . . connecting . . . intertwining . . . synchronizing. . . . There seems to be an endless exchange of body-mind-spirit elements of living and nonliving . . . happening without trying . . . releasing into it . . . letting it happen . . . the rhythm of your hands weaving in and out . . . threads blending . . . merging . . . in and out . . . beater packing threads . . . in and out. . . .

Just notice . . . being fully present in the moment . . . allowing the healing current to resonate in every cell of your beingness . . . new visions of healing emerging . . . inspirations coming. . . .

Sit with your healing tapestry. . . . What patterns have emerged? What emotions do you feel? What kind of energy is present for you? What about you is still in need of healing? What can you do to bring about that healing? Do you feel a connection with your work? Do you feel open to the inner wisdom gained from this process? What are the notes and melody of your healing song? What truths resonate within you . . . coming from your always present, inner, resonating, healing core?

Take a few energizing breaths . . . and as you come back into full awareness of the healing space within you . . . as you sit in your healing room . . . know that whatever is right for you at this point in time is unfolding . . . just as it should . . . and that you have done your best, regardless of the outcome.

With music still playing, invite students to continue the experience of creating their sacred work (30 minutes or longer). When the students have finished their sacred piece, have them attach their individual tapestry creations to the large blank tapestry. Suggest the following:

> With an awareness of a sense of sacredness, let yourself now attach your sacred creation onto the large blank tapestry with all the others. Feel the experience as you view the work of others with your own . . .

breathing deeply with each in breath. . . . With each out breath, an opportunity to release more . . . to feel gratitude and healing . . . for contributing to a master tapestry . . . for every thread you have touched . . . for every person and living and nonliving thing you have remembered . . . extending into and facilitating the healing process.

And now hear yourself sharing your healing work and the experience of contributing to a group tapestry with your colleagues . . . with others . . . being open . . . letting yourself be vulnerable . . . not judging . . . present in the moment . . . telling about your tapestry creation . . . sharing parts of your healing journey. . . .

## Appendix C

# Guidelines for Mindfulness Practice

What a wonderful opportunity to learn how to be present in the moment with the body, mind, and spirit. Healing happens in the present moment, not in the past or in the future. As we set aside time each day to practice mindfulness, we learn to recognize essential steps for healing. These are qualities such as softening, opening, receiving, forgiving, and feeling empathy, compassion, truth, and loving-kindness. There are many ways to begin your practice. You might use strategies such as relaxation, imagery, music, prayer, meditation, movement, or walking meditation. The following are some guidelines for beginning a practice of mindfulness:

- Set aside time each day to develop a practice of sitting mindfully for a minimum of 10 minutes.
- Find a quiet and comfortable place to practice.
- If your mind wanders and begins to attend to things that need to be done, places to go, unfinished business, or conversations with self or others, bring your mind back to the present moment. Some ways to do this are to focus on the breath, just observing the in breath and the out breath. You may wish to see each thought as it comes. In your mind, you may wish to place each thought on a leaf and see it flowing away in a stream of water. (Refer to Chapter 21 for more details on relaxation and mindfulness practice.)

You may find that you get bored with practice, cut it short, become uncomfortable, become angry, become restless, dislike certain emotions, or decide that nothing is happening. These are natural events as we learn to quiet the constant mind chatter or self-talk. Just approach your practice with a sense of exploring, opening, and lightening to the experience of being in the moment. Let go of any competitiveness or thought that there is a right way. If any uncomfortable emotions or memories come forward, you can either be with them for new insight or take a deep breath and open your eyes, and these experiences will leave. If you wish to delve into these uncomfortable emotions and feel stuck, you may wish to seek professional assistance from a nurse therapist or a counselor who specializes in a certain area, such as abuse work or loss/grief work.

As we learn to be in the moment, we access our natural wisdom. This occurs because we begin to notice the nature of our body, mind, and spirit when we create a state of intention and presence, recognizing new understanding and inner peace.

Appendix D

# Guidelines for Journaling

Journaling is a special process of recording events, thoughts, feelings, dreams, fears, losses, trauma or wounds, healing moments, and inner and external healing resources. There is no correct or right way to keep a journal. You may find that your journaling goes from structured writing to free-form writing with no structure. Read the discussion of journal keeping in Chapter 17. This chapter will also help you gain a deeper understanding of the journaling process and self-reflection.

You can write on a loose piece of blank or lined paper and keep these pages in a folder. However, when you choose a special notebook and writing pen or colored markers to record words and images, the process seems to take on a deeper significance. A few suggestions are offered:

- Set aside a minimum of 5 minutes a day to record in your journal outside of class.
- Find a quiet, comfortable place to journal.
- Bring your journal with you to each class. In each class session, different opportunities will be given to write in your journal following various experiential exercises.